ANIMAL SCIENCE, ISSUES AND PROFESSIONS

CANINE BEHAVIOR, CLASSIFICATION AND DISEASES

ANIMAL SCIENCE, ISSUES AND PROFESSIONS

Additional books in this series can be found on Nova's website under the Series tab.

Additional E-books in this series can be found on Nova's website under the E-book tab.

ANIMAL SCIENCE, ISSUES AND PROFESSIONS

CANINE BEHAVIOR, CLASSIFICATION AND DISEASES

ROBERTO LUIZ ANDRADE
AND
CRISTINA ISADORA BATISTA
EDITORS

Nova Science Publishers, Inc.
New York

For permission to use material from this book please contact us:
Telephone 631-231-7269; Fax 631-231-8175
Web Site: http://www.novapublishers.com

NOTICE TO THE READER

Library of Congress Cataloging-in-Publication Data

Canine behavior, classification and diseases / editors, Roberto Luiz Andrade and Cristina Isadora Batista.

p. cm.

Includes bibliographical references and index.

ISBN 978-1-62081-304-1 (hardcover)

1. Dogs--Diseases. 2. Dogs--Behavior. 3. Dogs--Classification. I. Andrade, Roberto Luiz. II. Batista, Cristina Isadora.

SF991.C233 2012

636.7--dc23

2012007378

Published by Nova Science Publishers, Inc. † New York

Contents

Preface

In this book, the authors gather current research in the study of canine behavior and diseases. Topics include galectin therapy in the treatment of canine mammary tumors; gene therapy for canine cancers; canine carcinogenesis as a valuable model for studying human cancers; parasitic zoonosis in dogs; dog bite injuries as a public health problem; and the genetics of dog behavior.

Chapter I – Canine mammary tumours (CMT) account for approximately 25-50% of all intact female dog tumours and 40-50% of affected animals develop malignant tumours. Despite CMT relevance, surgery remains the only effective treatment, which unfortunately is in many cases unsuccessful in preventing distant metastases, the main cause of CMT-related death. It is therefore necessary to understand the mechanisms underlying CMT metastasis, so that future therapeutic studies may be better targeted and thus more efficient. The metastatic process involves a series of events mediated by the balance between conflicting pro and anti adhesive forces. It is well-known that reversible steps of homotypic (cell-cell) and heterotypic (cell-ECM) adhesion are mediated in part by interactions between tumour cell surface glycan-receptors and their glycosylated ligands on other cells and/or within the tumour microenvironment. Galectins, a family of glycan-binding proteins, have been implicated in tumour progression and metastasis by influencing cell adhesion, angiogenesis, cell proliferation and apoptosis resistance. Galectin-1 and -3, well-studied members of this family, are believed to play opposing roles in several contexts. Our work has shown down-regulation of galectin-3 in primary malignant CMT and a concomitant decrease in galectin-3-binding-sites in the extracellular matrix (ECM). The decrease of galectin-3-binding sites in the tumour stroma was correlated with down-regulation of a β (1-O) galactosyltransferase, GLT25D1, crucial in collagen glycosylation, and concomitant up-regulation of stromal galectin-1. Stromal galectin-1 was accompanied by galectin-1 up-regulation in malignant CMT cells. In contrast, in intravascular tumour cells both anti-anoikis galectin-3 and its binding-sites were up-regulated in the cytoplasm and at the cell-surface while pro-anoikis galectin-1 was down-regulated and confined to the cell peri-nuclear region. Distant metastases however, expressed high levels of galectin-1 whereas galectin-3 was down-regulated. Thus, a role was envisioned for galectin-1 in growth and invasion at primary and distant sites and for galectin-3 in the systemic dissemination of tumour cells in malignant CMT. Moreover, our studies provided further evidence of the vital importance of glycosylation changes in modulating galectins function during malignant CMT systemic dissemination. Primary malignant CMT exhibited high contents of sialylated glycans compared to normal mammary tissues and removal of the sialic acid exposed galectin-3-binding sites in most tumour areas, although not in intravascular tumour cells which already expressed them. Mucins are very important glycan-carriers, aberrantly glycosylated and frequently sialylated in cancer. We showed that over-expression of MUC1 mucin is associated to distant metastases occurrence in malignant CMT. Interestingly, in intravascular tumour cells, but not in primary malignant CMT cells, there was physical interaction between galectin-3 and the un-sialylated form of the T antigen (Thomsen Friedenreich antigen), carried by MUC1. This interaction is believed to induce homotypic aggregation thus favouring blood-borne cell survival. Therefore there is a fine tuning of galectins function, both at their levels of expression, cellular and sub-cellular localization and at the availability of their glycan-ligands, which plays a crucial role in the development of distant metastases in malignant CMT. Galectin-inhibitors have been used with efficacy in several types of human cancer. Hence, galectins are valuable and exciting targets for new selective therapies in CMT.

Chapter II – Despite the important progress obtained in the treatment of some pets' malignancies, new treatments need to be developed. In this review we discuss the bases and we summarize the outcomes of published gene therapy veterinary clinical trials reported by many research centers up to date. A variety of tumors such as canine soft tissue sarcomas, osteosarcoma and lymphoma were subjected to different approaches. However, spontaneous canine melanoma (a highly aggressive tumor resistant to current therapies) was the preferred target. Both viral and mainly non-viral vectors as well as cytokine producing transgenic cells were used to deliver gene products as cytokines, suicide enzymes, xenogeneic tumor antigens, anti-angiogenic molecules and pro-apoptotic regulatory factors. Among other examples, we are presenting our own successful experience with suicide plus immunogene therapy for spontaneous canine melanomas and sarcomas. In general terms, very slight or no adverse collateral effects were found during this kind of treatments and usually treated patients displayed a better course of the disease (longer survival, delayed or suppressed local or systemic relapse, recovery of the quality of life), suggesting the utility of this sort of methodology as standard adjuvant treatment. The encouraging outcomes obtained in companion animals support their ready application in veterinary clinical oncology and serve as preclinical proof of concept and safety assay for future human gene therapy trials.

Chapter III – The biological complexity of human cancer has stimulated the development of complex experimental systems that could resemble in a natural and spontaneous manner the physiopathological aspects of cancer biology. Companion animals display many aspects of the complexity of human cancer filling the gap between *in vitro* and *in vivo* studies. Spontaneous tumors in dogs share a wide variety of epidemiological, biological and clinical features with human cancer, which makes this a valid tumor model system available for studying cancer biology in oncology research. In this review we summarize the importance of naturally occurring canine tumors as a valuable model for studying many aspects of human cancer, as well as the potential use of this animal model for the development of new cancer treatments.

Chapter IV – The dog can be involved in the mechanical transmission of infection by helminthes and protozoa; it has an epidemiological role in these zoonoses. The high rate of dogs naturally infected by endoparasites and the great possibility of acquiring this parasite justify the importance of attempting to prevent the occurrence of this illness. The aim of this paper is to demonstrate, through literature review, some clinical, epidemic and pathological aspects of endoparasite infection in the canine species.

Chapter V – Dog bites in humans are a public health problem of worldwide distribution. As a result of human population growth, the absence of responsible dog ownership polices and the increased numbers of free-roaming dogs especially in developing countries, dog bite injuries in people are frequently reported. The aim of this study was to determine the common regions of bites and to identify factors associated with dog bites in humans, in the city of Tuxtla Gutierrez, Chiapas, Mexico. A hospital-based questionnaire survey was conducted during 2007 among dog bites victims who visited a referral hospital (SSA) in the city of Tuxtla Gutierrez, Chiapas. A total of 194 persons were recorded. From those, 175 (89.7%) receive hospital care due to injuries caused by dog bites and 19 (10.3%) were attended by the bite of another domestic animal or wildlife species. Throughout the year, it was observed that the months with more cases of bites were mor frequently recorded during March and June matching with the official holiday periods in schools in Mexico. The age of persons attacked in a higher proportion (61.7%) were in the age groups of 1-10, 11-20 and 21-30 years old. There was no difference in the gender of the victims attacked by dogs (50.9 and 49.1% for male and female gender respectively). The dog bite victims occurred more commonly in people with low educational level (elementary and junior high school) in comparison with higher educational levels. Places where people were attacked by dogs were in the households and the streets, in most cases by stray dogs. In relation to the number of injuries caused by dog attacks, 80.9% of cases were reported as multiple lesions (type II) and only 19% had a single lesion associated with the attack (type I). The anatomic regions where victims were assaulted were in the legs, hands, feet and arms. From the dogs bitting people, 80.57% had owner and 19.4% were ownerless stray dogs. In addition to physical injuries, bites can potentially transmit a large number of zoonotic diseases (including rabies) to their victims. Increased educational awareness of people about the risk of dog bites is necessary together with enforcement of regulations for licensing of dogs, efficient stray dog population management and animal birth control programs to reduce bite incidents, especially in developing countries such as Mexico.

Chapter VI – All modern dog breeds are descendants of the grey wolf. Dogs were originally selected for behavioral traits: dogs have been bred to guard, herd, hunt, pull sledges, and to provide companionship. Early canid domestication involved selection for tameness. Studies of silver foxes at the Institute of Cytology and Genetics in Novosibirsk have shown that a few generations of selection for tameness can lead to a domesticated strain of foxes that not only show dog-like behaviors, but that also display phenotypic traits such as curly tails, drop ears, and loss of pigment. The early domestication of dogs was followed by the formation of dog breeds much later. Extreme founder effects, drift, and selection for novelty, in combination with genetic isolation during breed formation, have resulted in a canine genome sequence with features that are highly favorable for the molecular genetic study of inherited traits. Long linkage disequilibrium within breeds and a limited number of short common haplotypes across breeds greatly facilitate gene mapping. Canine genomic tools such as microarrays for genotyping and gene expression studies have enabled the identification of causal mutations for several canine morphological and disease susceptibility traits in recent years.

In this review chapter, we discuss the latest knowledge regarding the inheritance of behavioral traits in dogs. We also describe molecular genetic studies that have pinpointed some genetic variants that contribute to behavior. Behavioral traits that are discussed are canine personality, working behavior, anxiety, aggression, obsessive-compulsive disorder, and feeding behavior.

In: Canine Behavior, Classification and Diseases
Editors: R. L. Andrade and C. I. Batista
ISBN: 978-1-62081-304-1

Chapter I

Galectins - Potential Targets in Canine Mammary Tumour Therapy

***Joana T. de Oliveira*[1] *and Fátima Gärtner*[2]**
[1]Institute of Molecular Pathology and Immunology (IPATIMUP), University of Porto, Porto, Portugal
[2]Instituto de Ciências Biomédicas de Abel Salazar (ICBAS), University of Porto, Porto, Portugal

Abstract

Canine mammary tumours (CMT) account for approximately 25-50% of all intact female dog tumours and 40-50% of affected animals develop malignant tumours. Despite CMT relevance, surgery remains the only effective treatment, which unfortunately is in many cases unsuccessful in preventing distant metastases, the main cause of CMT-related death. It is therefore necessary to understand the mechanisms underlying CMT metastasis, so that future therapeutic studies may be better targeted and thus more efficient. The metastatic process involves a series of events mediated by the balance between conflicting pro and anti adhesive forces. It is well-known that reversible steps of homotypic (cell-cell) and heterotypic (cell-ECM) adhesion are mediated in part by interactions between tumour cell surface glycan-receptors and their glycosylated ligands on other cells and/or within the tumour microenvironment.

Galectins, a family of glycan-binding proteins, have been implicated in tumour progression and metastasis by influencing cell adhesion, angiogenesis, cell proliferation and apoptosis resistance. Galectin-1 and -3, well-studied members of this family, are believed to play opposing roles in several contexts. Our work has shown down-regulation of galectin-3 in primary malignant CMT and a concomitant decrease in galectin-3-binding-sites in the extracellular matrix (ECM). The decrease of galectin-3-binding sites in the tumour stroma was correlated with down-regulation of a β (1-O) galactosyltransferase, GLT25D1, crucial in collagen glycosylation, and concomitant up-regulation of stromal galectin-1. Stromal galectin-1 was accompanied by galectin-1 up-regulation in malignant CMT cells. In contrast, in intravascular tumour cells both anti-anoikis galectin-3 and its binding-sites were up-regulated in the cytoplasm and at the cell-surface while pro-anoikis galectin-1 was down-regulated and confined to the cell peri-nuclear region. Distant metastases however, expressed high levels of galectin-1 whereas galectin-3 was down-regulated. Thus, a role was envisioned for galectin-1 in growth and invasion at primary and distant sites and for galectin-3 in the systemic dissemination of tumour cells in malignant CMT.

Moreover, our studies provided further evidence of the vital importance of glycosylation changes in modulating galectins function during malignant CMT systemic dissemination. Primary malignant CMT exhibited high contents of sialylated glycans compared to normal mammary tissues and removal of the sialic acid exposed galectin-3-binding sites in most tumour areas, although not in intravascular tumour cells which already expressed them. Mucins are very important glycan-carriers, aberrantly glycosylated and frequently sialylated in cancer.

We showed that over-expression of MUC1 mucin is associated to distant metastases occurrence in malignant CMT. Interestingly, in intravascular tumour cells, but not in primary malignant CMT cells, there was physical interaction between galectin-3 and the un-sialylated form of the T antigen (Thomsen Friedenreich antigen), carried by MUC1. This interaction is believed to induce homotypic aggregation thus favouring blood-borne cell survival.

Therefore there is a fine tuning of galectins function, both at their levels of expression, cellular and sub-cellular localization and at the availability of their glycan-ligands, which plays a crucial role in the development of distant metastases in malignant CMT. Galectin-inhibitors have been used with efficacy in several types of human cancer. Hence, galectins are valuable and exciting targets for new selective therapies in CMT.

Introduction

General Concepts

During the last years pet animals life expectancy has been increasingly expanding, especially that of dogs and cats. As the population of aged animals increases so does the incidence of several types of tumours. Mammary gland tumours are the most prevalent in female dogs and have been studied for more than half a century. In spite of this, an effective treatment for this type of malignancy remains to be established.

Epidemiology

Canine mammary tumours (CMT) are the second most common type of canine neoplasia (25-50%), preceded only by skin tumours [1,2]. CMT are indeed the most frequent type of tumours in female dogs accounting for approximately 52% of all their tumours, up to approximately half of which being malignant [3,4]. Although CMT is a common condition of which the incidence is close to 205/100000 dogs per year [5], its incidence seems to be declining, due to the increased practice of ovariohysterectomy [4]. Indeed, in areas such as Southern Europe countries where ovariohisterectomy is less routinely performed the observed CMT incidence is somewhat higher [6]. Overall lifetime risk of CMT development in intact female dogs is up to 25% [7]. Regarding breed predisposition, Poodles, Cocker spaniels, Fox and Boston Terriers and Pointers appear to be at higher risk while mixed breed dogs reportedly have a lower incidence of CMT, resembling many other conditions with a possible strong genetic background [8,9].

No significant geographically related differences have been observed regarding CMT incidence [10,11,12]. Although it may appear at any age, CMT affects mainly elderly females, being uncommonly diagnosed before 2 to 4 years of age and presenting a higher incidence between 10 and 11 years [4,8].

Etiology

There are no clear and consensual risk factors for development of CMT. Female dogs presenting with pre-malignant CMT lesions are at increased risk of developing a malignant CMT later on in life [13,14]. Pseudopregnancy, gestation and giving birth at first stage, although debated, have not been associated to increased CMT development risk [4,15,16]. The practice of ovariohysterectomy, however, has been proved to confer a protective effect against the development of these tumours [12,17,18]. Despite that, there seems to be an age-related limit until which this effect can be observed. When the procedure is performed relatively late (around 4 years of age) the incidence resembles that observed for intact animals. On the other hand, in animals which underwent ovariohysterectomy before the first oestrous the incidence is drastically reduced with the risk of CMT development being estimated at 0.5%, increasing to 8% in animals spayed after the first oestrous and to 26% of the risk seen in intact animals, when the procedure is performed after the second oestrous [17,19]. Exogenous administration of progesterone derivatives for oestrus prevention has been associated to a greater risk of CMT development [20,21].

Concerning lifestyle, increased weight has been shown to be a risk factor to CMT development [22,23,24]. Diet, (high intake of red meat and low intake of chicken) seems also to be associated to increased risk of developing CMT [24].

Genetic factors have also been involved in CMT occurrence. BRCA1 and BRCA2 genes, of which inherited mutations confer a 56-84% lifetime risk of breast cancer development [25,26], appear to be related to CMT development [27]. Although not associated to overall CMT risk, animals carrying the COMT G482A polymorphism variant allele have a threefold likelihood of developing mammary tumors after 9 years of age when compared to non-carriers [28]. No other studied risk factors have been proven to be related to CMT occurrence.

Physiopathology

The hormonal microenvironment, where progestagens are known to favour epithelial and myoepithelial hyperplasia inducing lobulo-alveolar development while estradiol stimulates ductal growth consensually influences the development of CMT [3,29,30]. As such, repeated oestrus cycles gradually prime the mammary gland for CMT development [15]. Malignant CMT appear to progress from benign CMT [31]. Despite the fact that both normal and neoplastic glands showing ER (estrogen receptor) and PR (progestagen receptor) expression [32,33], the levels of expression seem to vary. Benign CMT present higher ER expression when compared to their malignant counterparts [32,34], and higher PR expression levels are also observed in benign when compared to malignant CMT [34].

Even though 4 or 6 pairs may be observed, most female dogs present five pairs of mammary glands. However, approximately 65 to 70% of all CMT develop in the caudal abdominal and inguinal ones [3]. The reason for this preferential localization site for CMT development is still unknown but may be related to their increased volume and proliferative alterations in response to the local hormonal microenvironment [3,30]. It has been suggested that caudal glands maintain secretory activity longer than cranial ones being therefore more prone to CMT development [12]. Further corroborating an association between microenvironment and CMT occurrence, 50-70% of affected animals present more than one nodule, of different histological types in distinct mammary glands [12,17,35]. Further evidence for a multifocal origin comes from the observation of different stem lines recognized by a different DNA index as measured by flow cytometry [36] However the possibility of malignant tumour cells being seeded in different glands by lymph vessels [37] or by way of small veins which cross the midline together with craniocaudal anastomoses cannot be ruled out [38]. Moreover, in this regard, neoplastic glands present more lymphatic anastomoses when compared to normal ones [39].

Metastasis

Metastasis, tumour spread from the site of a primary growth to distant target organs, is the main cause of cancer-related morbidity and mortality, in female dogs bearing malignant CMT and its prevention and or treatment after development remain unquestionably the major clinical challenge associated with this malignancy.

CMT metastasis occurs *via* lymphatic vessels or *via* blood vessels, the first being the most frequently observed. Since lymph drainage from mammary glands goes to the axillary and inguinal lymph nodes and sometimes prescapulary nodes, these should be systematically assessed for the presence of metastases. The lungs are the most frequent target organs despite others such as liver, bone, brain, etc. have also been reported [35].

The development of metastases is a complex process engaging many steps [40]. During progression tumour cells which are able to detach from primary tumour masses and travel to distant sites may succeed in founding new implants, depending on a complex series of coordinated events [40,41]. The tumour microenvironment plays a major influence on the behaviour of tumour cells which, under particular stimuli, such as hypoxia, tend to cross the tissue underlying the malignant growth in order to expand and invade new sites. Moreover, the same *de novo* formed vessels, by angiogenesis due to hypoxia, will not only support the primary growth but also provide an escape route for invading cells which through intravasation will access the circulation. A metastasis favourable microenvironment is, both at primary and secondary sites, dependent on the active crosstalk between tumour stroma, which includes inflammatory and endothelial cells as well as fibroblasts and the extracellular matrix, and tumour cells themselves [42]. Data from CMT specimens and malignant CMT cell lines have pointed to a fundamental role of galectins 1 and 3 and their ligands in the process of vessel invasion and blood-borne survival as well as primary and secondary site tumour growth [43,44,45].

Diagnosis

Pain and /or discomfort are not typical symptoms of CMT and most early malignant CMT are asymptomatic. Hence CMT are often first felt by owners or clinicians during routine check-ups and most dogs appear healthy at time of presentation [12]. The general approach to evaluation of CMT includes complete patient history, physical examination, and complementary diagnostic means, such as thoracic radiographs, abdominal ultrasound and blood examination. . Important history data include age, spaying status, age at ovariohisterectomy if spayed, reproductive cycles, lactation and progesterone administration. Elderly intact females which have undergone multiple oestrus cycles or which have been administered progestagens in order to avoid them are more likely to present CMT. During physical examination a thorough exam of both mammary gland chains and regional lymph nodes, which may be felt when enlarged, must be performed [12,35]. Needle cytology may aid in differentiating other causes of mammary masses from mammary neoplasia and in identifying non-mammary gland derived tumours. Improved cytology specimen collection of the lesions with at least 4 samples taken *per* mass increases the accuracy of the diagnosis and agreement with later histopathological analysis [46,47].

Non-imaging approach include haematological and biochemical profiles which although not presenting specific alterations in CMT are important to identify concurrent geriatric diseases, paraneoplastic syndromes, coagulation disorders, common in advanced stages of this condition, and to assess the anaesthetic risk before surgery [48].

Imaging approaches are crucial in order to assess the presence of distant metastases and include thoracic radiographs, CT (computerized tomography) [49] and abdominal ultrasound [12].

Animals with metastatic disease may show systemic symptoms, the severity of which is dependent on both the amount and location of metastases. Symptoms include lethargy, weight loss, cough, dyspnea, lymphoedema, fatigue and lameness [35].

Differential Diagnosis

Mammary masses may be broadly classified as benign or malignant. Common benign mammary masses include hyperplasia and abscesses. Pain not being characteristic of CMT, when present, may suggest the alternative diagnosis of an inflammatory process. Ultrasound may reveal cystic structures which can be simple or complex. An image with uneasily defined walls and a hypoecoic centre should raise the suspicion of an abscess which may be confirmed as mentioned by cytology. Definite CMT diagnosis is based on histopathological assessment, which remains the gold standard method for the diagnosis of this condition.

Histological Types and Grading

Several different systems have been used to classify the CMT lesions in an attempt to predict their clinical behaviour. The importance of the WHO classification for mammary tumours in for domestic animals is underlined by its frequent adoption.

Table 1 summarizes the different types of malignant CMT described [50]. Nevertheless, the histological classification of CMT used in Veterinary Medicine is not completely uniform and lacks molecular basis which could contribute to better assessment of both prognosis and treatment options. Grading of CMT has also been performed using different methods, being the modified Elston and Ellis method, frequently applied [51,52,53]. A new classification of CMT resembling the sub-grouping used in human breast cancer into Luminal A and B, HER+, Basal-like and non classified or Normal-like, based on the expression of markers such as ER, PR,HER2,CK5 has been attempted. The objective is to improve knowledge of metastatic potential and thus prognosis accuracy as well as to implement specific targeted therapy, however there is controversy regarding its usefulness [32,54].

Table 1. WHO histological classification for malignant CMT (adapted from Misdorp et al., 1999)

Malignant CMT	
In situ carcinoma	
Complex carcinoma	
Simple carcinoma	
	Tubulopapillary carcinoma
	Solid carcinoma
	Anaplastic carcinoma
Special types of carcinomas	
	Spindle cell carcinomas
	Squamous cell carcinoma
	Mucinous carcinoma
	Lipid-rich carcinoma
Carcinosarcoma	
Carcinosarcoma or sarcoma in benign tumour	
Sarcoma	
	Fibrosarcoma
	Osteosarcoma
	Other sarcomas

Staging

In addition to the above mentioned histological classification, the WHO also suggests a TNM (tumour-node-metastases) staging method which attempts to provide more clinically useful prognostic information [3] and allows better comparison beyond tumour burden, which may be essential when evaluating the efficacy of new treatments. The staging system is described in table 2. It is noteworthy that the higher the stage, the poorer the prognosis. Yet, the need to arrive at a better staging system has been stressed recently [55].

Treatment

Despite its frequently aggressive behaviour and distant metastases development, prognosis assessment and treatment for CMT are often inadequate.

Table 2. Modified TNM staging of malignant CMT

Stage	PrimaryTumor	Regional LN Status	Distant Metastases
I	T1	NO	MO
II	T2	NO	MO
III	T3	NO	MO
IV	Any T	N1	MO
V	Any T	Any N	M1

T1 < 3 cm maximum diameter.
T2 3-5 cm maximum diameter.
T3 > 5 cm maximum diameter.
NO Histologically no metastasis.
N1 Histologically observed metastasis.
MO No distant metastases.
M1 Detection of distant metastases.

Surgery

Surgery is considered primary treatment for malignant CMT. Many patients with early-stage malignant CMT may be cured with surgery alone provided that the margins are clean and the tumour has not already invaded [48]. However this is not always the case and approximately 50% of the animals already have either micrometastases or well-established metastases at the time of surgery [35]. Several different surgical techniques were described; nevertheless, radical removal of the ipsilateral chain has been recently advised due to a 58% probability of new homolateral CMT development observed in a prospective study, using a more conservative technique [56]. Routine removal of the lymph nodes is advisable and often performed on the superficial inguinal nodes however, due to close proximity to the brachial plexus, the proper axillary lymph nodes are not commonly resected [35]. It is a well-established fact that cure probability and general success of oncologic surgery is highly dependent on surgical volume and surgeon experience [57]. Although the vast majority of dogs affected by mammary tumours are subjected to mastectomy at a potentially curable stage, effective post-operative protocols aiming to prevent and /or delay metastases development have not yet been devised. This stems mainly from lack of knowledge in the field of CMT pathophysiology which in turn precludes the use of its involved molecules as dependable cancer typing and staging markers.

Research in CMT Adjuvant Therapy

Adjuvant treatment of human breast cancer is designed to treat micrometastatic disease, or human breast cancer cells that have escaped the primary tumour site and regional lymph nodes but which have still not given rise to clinically detectable metastases. Over the last 2 decades, research on human breast cancer has provided overwhelming knowledge of the disease, ensuing more efficient and less morbid treatments. Adjuvant therapy has been estimated to reduce up to 72% the mortality rate of human breast cancer [58]. Reference! However in malignant CMT, improvements in prevention of recurrence by post-operative adjuvant therapies have been poor.

Clinical trials, attempting adjuvant chemotherapeutic protocols for malignant CMT have shown to be mostly uneffective. Antimetabolites such as 5-fluorouracil (5FU), gemcitabine and methrotexate have been used in combination regimens for breast cancer. Gemcitabine targets the ribonucleotide reductase and as fluorouracil leads to tumour cell apoptosis. In a recent study, dogs treated with surgery alone or surgery followed by gemcitabine showed no significant differences in time to local recurrence, time to distant metastases and overall survival (OS) [59]. 5FU is a pyrimidine analogue which inhibits thymidylate synthase. Real alkylating agents, such as cyclophosphamide, attach an alkyl group to DNA of fast proliferating cells, thereby being cytotoxic. Indeed Yamashita et al indicated effects of such compounds in experimental settings of xenografted CMT in mice [60], and benefit of adjuvant therapy combining 5FU with cyclophosphamide was reported in a small series of malignant CMT [61]. However, more accurate studies are warranted in order to fully state the benefit of using this combination in CMT therapy.

Other agents such as cisplatin and carboplatin induce DNA damage and are thus sometimes referred as alkylating-like. Carboplatin is used in breast cancer combined therapy, while cisplatin is not used routinely for breast cancer treatment, but has been recently suggested to induce an effective response in a subset of patients with Triple-Negative Breast Cancer [62].

Taxanes block cell division by preventing microtubule formation. Despite a few conflicting studies, taxanes are among the most active and commonly used agents in human early-breast cancer therapy, with both doxetacel and paclitaxel being applied [63,64]. However, in a small prospective study the combination of doxetacel and cyclosporin A did not induce responses in malignant CMT [65], while another study assessing the efficacy and toxicity of paclitaxel noticed only 20% partial responses with high toxicity reported [66]. Docetaxel, another taxane, also failed to demonstrate efficacy in CMT [67]. Thus, the use of taxanes alone in malignant CMT treatment does not seem effective.

Anthracycline-based regimens have been used in the treatment of early-stage breast cancer for decades. Anthracyclines such as epirubicin and doxorubicin inhibit topoisomerase IIa (TOP2A), and are thus particularly useful in cases presenting with TOP2A and HER2 amplification [68]. Doxorubicin has been included in several protocols of adjuvant therapy for human breast cancer, including stage III and locally advanced breast cancer [69]. However, doxorubicin [67] failed to demonstrate efficacy in CMT.

The common expression of drug resistance proteins in CMT may provide an explanation for the relative poor efficacy of cytostatics [70].

Regarding adjuvant hormone therapy, tamoxifen is a selective ER modulator (SERM) which inhibits ER signalling in the mammary gland. It has been approved for human breast cancer treatment since the early 1980's and was shown to reduce the relative risk of distant, ipsilateral and contralateral breast cancer recurrence by up to 50% in tumours with high ER expression [71]. *In vitro* studies have shown CMT cells to be sensitive to tamoxifen [72]. Nonetheless, its oestrogenic side effects impair tamoxifen use in clinical trials in dogs [73]. Thus, as an alternative ovariohysterectomy could be an option for reducing hormonal influence in CMT spreading. Nevertheless, studies have not shown consensual effects of pre-, peri- or post-operative spaying on the progression of malignant CMT [74-77]. A study limited only to hormonal receptor positive tumours would be of better use to study the benefits of hormonal withdrawal in such CMT cases. Aglepristone, a progesterone antagonist, treatment has also been recently studied and showed a potential to decrease the proliferation index of PR-positive CMT in a small number of animals although no association to disease progression was evaluated [78]. Regarding other hormonal therapies, a study in a small number of animals yielded promising results with a relapse-free survival of 88% at 2 years in animals treated with goserelin, a LHRH agonist [79]. Based on a probable microvasculature tightening effect, pre- and post- surgical intravenous administration of desmopressin has shown to inhibit lymph node and lung metastases and significantly increase DFS and OS in females dogs bearing CMT [80,81]. However, due to the low number of animals used in these studies larger scaled ones are warranted. The present situation leads to the absence of meaningful clinical trials and hence established adjuvant therapies.

In targeted chemotherapy for human metastatic breast cancer, besides the above described agents, vinorelbine a vinca alkaloid has been more recently advocated with overall response rates of 35-45%. In a dosage-finding study, 2 dogs with metastatic bronchoalveolar carcinoma experienced a partial response for an overall response rate of 12.5% in 16 dogs with gross measurable disease [82]. In a phase II clinical trial in dogs with cutaneous mast cell tumors vinorelbine was associated with an overall response rate of 13% [83]. No study has been so far performed with vinorelbine in dogs bearing CMT. An ongoing phase III trial is currently evaluating the role of zoledronic acid in the adjuvant therapy of women with stage II/III breast cancer [84]. Despite having been reported its possible usefulness in canine osteosarcoma [85], no study has been so far performed regarding its efficacy against CMT.

Present knowledge of carcinogenesis and metastases shows great similarity between human and canine mammary cancer. The widely differing clinical results obtained in malignant CMT trials with chemotherapeutic agents, compared to humans, can thus be most probably due to insufficient patient number for correct trial design. But above all it seems that only a parallel subtyping and respective comparison will elicit dependable scientific evidence. In Veterinary Oncology both *in vitro* and *in vivo* studies should take into account molecule expression patterns of the tumours, allowing the sub grouping of animals by tumour type and also considering prognostic and predictive factors. This would aid in better understanding therapy response in clinical trials and substantiate the use of combined targeted therapies.

Prognosis

Prognostic factors may be divided into clinical and histopathological factors.

Clinical Factors

Increased tumour size or volume are reported to be related to lower survival and shorter disease-free interval (DFI) by most studies [86-88]. Ulceration was significantly associated to survival and shorter DFI [86,89,90]. The presence of multiple malignant CMT was significantly associated to DFI [86,90]. Tumour fixation to underlying tissue was significantly associated to lower survival [88]. Presence of lymph node metastases have been significantly associated to lower survival and shorter DFI [86,88,89]. Distant metastases are as expected significantly related to poorer survival [76,86]. Surgical technique was also found to influence prognosis since incomplete excision as assessed by the status of the surgical margin is significantly related to lower survival [23]. The animal reproductive status, early age at first estrous was associated with higher disease-free survival (DFS) [86,90]. On the other hand, short estrous duration and decreased number of oestrus cycles were associated to lower survival and shorter DFI [86]. Dogs neutered at the time of surgery were more likely to survive 2 years after surgery than dogs which were subjected to the procedure [87]. However, negative effects of ovariectomy overall on survival in dogs with CMT reported by others [74,75,77] suggest that since most metastatic tumours are negative to steroid receptors [32], a positive effect of spaying would be restricted to animals bearing receptor positive tumours. Regarding age, while other conflicting studies exist, older age was significantly associated to poorer survival and DFI [86,89,90]. Obesity was found not to influence survival of dogs bearing CMT [77]. Interestingly, malignant CMT-bearing dogs fed with low fat diet and high protein content presented a significantly increased median survival time [23].

Histological Factors

Factors such as histological type have also been associated to prognosis. Although uncommon in dogs, sarcomas (11,2%) are significantly associated to poorer survival [87,89,91]. Carcinosarcomas have also been associated to poor survival when compared to non-mixed malignant tumours [74]. Within carcinomas, the complex type seems to be associated to better survival than the simple one [74,91]. Histological invasion of the surrounding stroma has been associated to poorer survival [23,91] as has vascular invasion which was significantly associated to decreased survival at 12 and 24 months after surgery [92]. Poorly differentiated tumours (grade III) have a 7 fold increased risk of death 24 months after surgery when compared to moderately differentiated ones (grade II), this rises to a 21 fold increase when compared to grade II and well-differentiated tumours (grade I) [93]. Tumours with mitotic indexes above 3.09 were significantly associated to poor survival both at 12 and 24 months after surgery [92]. ER- and/or PR-positive tumours were suggested to present a better prognosis, possibly because of an association with a more common complex type [94]. DNA ploidy and S-phase rate were significantly related to increased relative hazards [89]. Altogether, these may be important features in deciding on a course of treatment for CMT when available.

New Prognostic Assessment

Several important attempts have been done in order to establish new prognostic markers by molecular studies such as: detection of circulating tumor cells (CTC) which had a proven prognostic value for human breast cancer [95]; refined search for micrometastases presence using immunohistochemistry [55]; p53 gene mutations which appear to be associated to CMT-related death [96]; 2 recognized single nucleotide polymorphisms in the Catechol-O-methyltransferase (COMT) gene (COMTG216A and COMTG482A) which when simultaneously present are associated to local CMT recurrence [97]; tumour proliferative rates, assessed with MIB-1 labelling indices which have been associated to metastases occurrence [98], DFS [86] and overall survival (OS) [92]; Caveolin-1-positive CMT which strongly correlated to shorter OS [99]; Cox-2 overexpression which was associated to shorter survival time [100]; E-cadherin and beta-catenin reduced expression which were significantly associated with shorter OS and DFS [101] as well as other factors of poor prognosis [102]; MUC1 mucin over-expression which is significantly associated to distant metastases occurrence [52]; TIMP-2 of which increased expression was significantly associated to development of distant metastases, lower OS and lower DFS [103]; and uPA of which high stromal expression was significantly associated with development of distant metastases, lower OS and DFS [104].

These factors might be evaluated as valuable parameters which can be associated to classical prognostic features in order to aid the clinical decision for treatment in the manner of Human Medicine's ongoing approach.

Future Perspectives

As mentioned above, efforts have been done concerning adjuvant therapeutic clinical trials in malignant CMT [59,60,67] but yielded conflicting results, mostly with no significant influence in the outcome of affected animals. Hence, the search for effective post-operative adjuvant chemotherapeutic protocols for CMT remains an exciting field in veterinary oncology research. Consequently, it is crucial to better understand the pathophysiological mechanisms underlying the aggressive capacity of CMT.

In this regard, recently, a family of animal lectins, galectins, has been reported to play paramount functions in different steps of the metastatic process in malignant CMT. They could thus be of potential therapeutic use in combined adjuvant therapies [43]. Galectin-1 and -3, the most studied galectins, are involved in normal cell adhesion, migration and tissue remodeling during mammal development and regeneration processes [105]. Galectins display a high degree of redundancy in their functions and the elimination of a specific galectin from a model system has not proved to severely affect it [105]. Galectin-1 knock-out mice display only defects in olfactory axon pathfinding [106] while galectin-3 knock-outs present defects in neutrophil accumulation during inflammation [107]. Therefore, galectin-inhibitors able to act upon several members of this family would most likely be effective to impair metastatic tumour spread. Galectin-3 natural ligands such as galactose, lactose, polylactosamine and N-acetyllactosamine (LacNac) were identified [108] and are considered as natural inhibitors [109-111]. Pectins, from various dietary sources have also shown enhanced galectin inhibition related to higher arabinose and galactose contents suggesting the importance of arabinogalactans in inhibiting galectin-3-mediated cellular interactions [112]. These data rapidly lead to the enthusiastic exploration of galectins as therapeutic targets in cancer. Several studies pointed to anti-liver metastases activity of arabinogalactans [113,114] and anti-proliferative and pro-apoptotic actions of okra pectin on melanoma cells through galectin-3 interactions [115]. Moreover, many other studies have shown anti-metastatic properties of the galectin-inhibiting Modified Citrus Pectin (MCP). Furthermore, high-affinity carbohydrate-based galectin-3 inhibitors have been developed through the production of LacNac [110] and galactose [116] derivatives. Galectin-3 synthetic inhibitor lactulosyl-L-leucine (Lac-L-Leu) reduced the number of established breast cancer cells (MDA-MB-435Lung2) pulmonary metastases and Lac-L-Leu/paclitaxel combination decreased both the number and the incidence of pulmonary metastases [117]. As an alternative to sugar based inhibitors, artificial peptide inhibitors have also been used and found to be effective in preventing binding of several galectins [118]. These peptide based inhibitors were found to inhibit metastasis-associated cell adhesion [119]. In order to better understand where and how galectin-innhibitors could impair tumour cells as they go through the malignant CMT metastatic cascade, critical rate-limiting steps in the metastatic process mediated by β-galactoside-galectin interactions and reports of their inhibition in other cancer types will be discussed bellow.

One of the determining factors in tumour progression is the immunologic system. On the one hand, immune-surveillance mechanisms reduce tumour incidence [120]. On the other hand, immune-related mechanisms have been found to promote tumour progression [121]. Galectins were found to be expressed by several immune cells in CMT [43] and are known to regulate their functions [122]. Adding to that, tumour cells themselves release galectins both positively and negatively modulating the immune response. Indeed, the amount of galectin-1 secreted by different tumour cell types is sufficient to induce T cell death when it is released in the ECM [123]. Moreover, galectin-1 was elegantly linked to immune privilege by modulating survival or polarization of effector T cells [124]. Inhibition of galectin-1 gene expression was found to arrest tumour growth, further confirming a growth-promoting activity of endogenous galectin-1 [125]. Furthermore, galectin-1 expression in primary CMT was significantly associated to increased tumour size [45].

Regarding angiogenesis, when compared to vessels in normal tissue, the tumour vasculature is highly disorganized with tortuous and leaky vessels presenting irregular and thin vessel walls [40]. These neovessels not only support primary tumour growth but also provide a route to distant sites since their above described characteristics make them more prone to be invaded than normal vessels [40]. Angiogenesis switch on/off is dependent on pro- and anti-angiogenic molecules which may arise from tumour, endothelial and stromal cells, as well as from the extracellular matrix (ECM) [126]. Tumour-associated hypoxia activates the hypoxia-inducible factor (HIF1alpha) [127] which induces expression of pro-angiogenic factors among which VEGF [128] as well as galectin- 1 and -3 [129]. It is of note that pro-angiogenic galectin-1 is up-regulated in primary malignant CMT [45]. Adding to that, cells surrounding necrotic areas strongly expressed both galectin-1 [45] and -3 [43] in CMT and CMT xenografts, further suggesting a role in response to hypoxia in these tumours. Galectin-3 is a potent angiogenic factor shown to be intimately involved in endothelial cell morphogenesis and angiogenesis. It acts as a chemoattractant for endothelial cells and induces endothelial cell motility, invasion through matrigel and capillary tube formation [130-132]. Moreover, expression of VEGF was ubiquitously found in normal and malignant canine mammary tissues [53]. Given that galectin-3 is an important mediator of VEGF-mediated angiogenic response [130] and it is found to be expressed by hypoxia-exposed subpopulations in primary malignant CMT [43], this further suggests a role of the lectin in angiogenesis of these tumours. Galectin3-inhibitors impair its angiogenic activity by blocking chemotaxis of human endothelial cells and by inhibiting *in vitro* capillary tube formation by endothelial cells both in a dose-dependent manner [132]. Moreover, galectin-3 pro-angiogenic function was found to be inhibited by MCP in breast cancer xenografts [131]. Thus, it might have the same anti-angiogenic effect in CMT.

Next to the escape from primary sites and vessel intravasation, blood-borne tumour cells need to survive the type of apoptosis associated with the loss of anchorage (anoikis) and a journey through the circulation. Despite a general decrease in galectin-3 expression in primary malignant CMT, interestingly, intravascular tumour cells over-express this galectin [43]. Galectin-3 has been shown to protect tumour cells from anoikis [133,134] by regulating their transition through the cell cycle, inducing a cell cycle arrest at an anoikis-insensitive point (late G1 phase) [133]. Adding to a predominant up-regulation of anti-anoikis galectin-3 at the cell surface and in the cytoplasm of malignant CMT intravascular cells, pro-anoikis galectin-1 was down-regulated when compared to sedentary cells [45]. Interestingly, galectin-3 is an endogenous competitor of the pro-anoikis effector galectin-1 in cancer [135]. Moreover, galectin-3 further contributes to anoikis survival by interacting with tumour-associated antigen, Thomsen-Friedenreich antigen (T antigen) which induces tumour cell homotypic aggregation inside vessels [136]. Notably, vessel-invading cells of malignant CMT also present physical interactions between galectin-3 and the T antigen [44].

After tumour cells lodge in target organ microvessels, they can either proliferate intravascularly, until metastatic tumour outgrows blood vessel and invades distant organ parenchyma [137] or extravasate before initiating a secondary tumour growth. The following rate-limiting step in metastasis is thus dependent on tumour cell arrest in distant organ microvasculature. Galectin-3 mediates metastatic cell adhesion to the endothelium. [138-140]. Further, it appears that galectin-3 interactions with T antigen mediate also the initial adhesion of tumour cells to endothelial cells at the sites of primary attachment to the endothelium, and this is dependent on decreased sialylation of the antigen [141]. In malignant CMT not only expression of galectin-3-binding sites was detected in endothelium but also focal expression of these binding sites was detected in intravascular tumour cells [43] while in sedentary cells these seem to be masked by sialic acid both in CMT and CMT-U27 xenografts [44]. Several studies converged) demonstrating galectin-3's role in metastases in experimental settings. Both tumour cell-endothelium adhesion and tumour cell homotypic adhesion were shown to be galectin-3 dependent in mouse melanoma and rat prostate cancer cell lines through the lectin's inhibition with MCP [142,143]. Furthermore, a dose-dependent inhibition of breast cancer cells' adhesion to human endothelial cells in vitro was demonstrated using the same galectin-3 inhibitor [131].

The process of extravasation from vessels involves a series of tumour cell interactions with the extracellular matrix (ECM) proteins present on basement membranes and target organ stroma. Malignant CMT displayed an overall loss of galectin-3-binding sites in the ECM. Loss of galectin-3-binding sites was correlated with an overall decrease in galactosylation of the ECM, down-regulation of GLT25D1, a β (1-O) galactosyltransferase that modifies collagen [43]. Moreover, the occupancy of galectin-3-binding sites by other endogenous galectins was also observed with an up-regulation of stromal galectin-1 and to a lesser extent of cleaved galectin-3 [43]. That tumour cell-ECM proteins such as laminin interaction are mediated by galectin-3 was clearly demonstrated through its inhibition by MCP [144]. As galectin-3, galectin-1 is also able to both stimulate and inhibit cellular adhesion through cross-linking glycans on integrins and through binding to laminin impeding integrins' accessibility, respectively [145]. Moreover, galectin-1 increases the adhesion of cancer cell lines to the ECM [146]. In addition, galectin-1 promotes increased cancer cell motility *in vitro* [147]. Galectin-inhibitors, citrus pectin polysaccharides were reported to impair invasion through matrigel of human metastatic breast carcinoma cells, in a dose-dependent manner [148]. Thus, *in vivo* effects of galectin-inhibitors on experimental metastasis of various malignancies may involve inhibition of tumour cell invasion.

Following the initial arrest in distant organs and extravasation, most tumour cells suffer apoptosis induced by several stimuli, and less than 2% survive giving rise to micrometastases [40]. This is therefore, one of the most important rate-limiting steps in the efficiency of the metastatic process. Galectin-3 present in the cytoplasm, regulates tumour cell apoptosis, mainly by acting upon key mitochondrial apoptotic pathways, [149] thus potentially playing a significant role in early tumour cell survival in target organs. On the other hand, nuclear located galectin-3 inhibited metastasis, anchorage independence and promoted apoptosis [150]. Malignant CMT tumours exhibited a statistically significant decrease of nuclear galectin-3 expression with the majority of the immunostaining confined to the cytoplasm as did distant metastases [43]. This anti-apoptotic function of galectin-3 could be targeted by galectin-inhibitors [149].

In order for micrometastases to evolve into clinically relevant secondary tumours, beyond 1mm, neo vascular supply is crucial. Then chemotaxis to endothelial cells and the development of new blood vessels occurring by angiogenesis constitutes the next vital step. Distant metastases expressed even stronger levels of pro-angiogenic galectin-1 expression when compared to primary malignant CMT [45]. In the same well-established CMT metastatic lesions galectin-3 is over-expressed surrounding necrotic areas [43]. A statistically significant decrease in angiogenesis and spontaneous metastasis of breast cancer xenografts was observed in animals treated with galectin-inhibitors [131]. Therapy targeting angiogenesis is regarded as one of the most promising and important targets in cancer therapy.

Most anti-neoplastic drugs act by tumour cell apoptosis induction *via* the mitochondrial apoptotic pathway [151]. Galectin-3 impairs this pathway, [149] and has been shown to directly regulate the sensitivity of tumour cells to several chemotherapeutic agents such as cisplatin [152], staurosporine [153], etoposide [154], bortezomib [154], dexamethasone, [155] and doxorubicin [156]. Galectin-3 inhibitors might sensitize tumour cells to cytotoxic drugs by inhibiting galectin-3 anti-apoptotic effects. Galectin-3-inhibitors have so far been proven to reverse multiple myeloma cell resistance to bortezomib and to enhance their response to apoptosis induced by dexamethasone [155] and treatment of hemangiosarcoma cells with galectin-3 inhibitor increased their sensitivity to doxorubicin-induced apoptosis [156]. Thus, addition of galectin-3-inhibitors to therapeutic regimens for treating CMT could have the potential to improve the effects of chemotherapy. In addition to enhancing apoptosis induced by cytotoxic drugs, galectin-3 inhibitors may be able themselves to induce apoptosis [152,155] in tumour cells as suggested by multiple myeloma cells in which MCP induced apoptosis through a caspase-8-to-caspase-3 signalling cascade and the effect of several forms of citrus pectin on apoptosis induction in human prostate cancer cells [157].

Galectin-inhibitors were shown to be effective experimentally either *in vitro* or *in vivo*, or both, against prostate carcinoma [157], colon carcinoma [158], breast carcinoma [131], melanoma [142], multiple myeloma [155], and hemangiosarcoma [156]. Moreover, galectin-inhibitors usefulness has been suggested to enhance the effects of doxorubicin, the currently standard of care for dogs bearing hemangiosarcoma [156]. The specific binding between a pectin-derived galactan and recombinant human galectin-3 was demonstrated supporting the suggested molecular hypothesis for the anticancer action of MCP by demonstrating that bioactive fragments from pectin can bind specifically to galectin-3 [159]. Fluorescently labeled galactan binding to a highly metastatic CMT cell line was evaluated with and without shRNA inhibition of galectin-3 and demonstrated a strongly decreased binding upon galectin-3 silencing (de Oliveira et al. Unpublished data). This points to galectin-3 as the main glycan-receptor responsible for galactan binding to CMT-U27, although not completely excluding binding to other endogenous galectins, and thus supports the use of pectins in metastatic targeting combined therapies in malignant CMT.

Conclusion

In conclusion, increased owner awareness and improving Veterinary care has been leading to earlier diagnosis at stages amenable to complete surgical resection of CMT. Consequently, survival rates to the condition but also late onset metastases are expected to slowly increase. The use of adjuvant therapies that would significantly aid in further ameliorating survival chances of patients with CMT is in its primordium and thus the fundamental interest in understanding CMT progression at the molecular level. Due to galectins' adhesive, angiogenic and apoptosis-related properties, they are involved in multiple CMT critical rate-limiting metastatic steps. By inhibiting galectin-3 functions and enhancing apoptosis induced by cytotoxic drugs, galectin-inhibitors hold the potential to increase dramatically the efficiency of adjuvant chemotherapy in CMT. Galectin-inhibitors were shown to be effective experimentally against several types of cancer. Human clinical studies performed to date demonstrated that galectin-inhibitors significantly increased prostate specific antigen doubling time in patients with recurrent prostate cancer [160] thus confirming its foreseen usefulness in treating spontaneous cancer. Thus, galectin-inhibition is promising in co-adjuvant treatment in CMT as it is in multiple other human and canine malignancies.

References

[1] Fidler IJ, Brodey RS. The biological behavior of canine mammary neoplasms. *J. Am. Vet. Med. Assoc.* 1967 Nov 15;151(10):1311-8.

[2] Moulton JE (1990) Tumors of the Mammary Gland. In Moulton JE (ed): *Tumors in Domestic Animals*, 3rd ed. University of California Press, pp 518-550.

[3] Rutteman GR, Withrow SJ, MacEwen EG (2001) Tumours of the Mammary Gland. In Withrow SJ, MacEwen EG (eds): Small Animal Clinical Oncology, 3rd ed., W. B. *Saunders Company*, pp 455-477.

[4] Schneider R (1970) Comparison of age, sex and incidence rations in human and canine breast cancer. *Cancer* 26, 4119-4126.

[5] Dobson JM, Samuel S, Milstein H, Rogers K, Wood JLN (2002) Canine neoplasia in the UK: estimates of incidence rates from a population of insured dogs. *J. Small An. Pract.* 43, 240-246.

[6] Perez Alenza MD, Peña L, del Castillo N, Nieto AI.Factors influencing the incidence and prognosis of canine mammary tumours.*J. Small Anim. Pract.* 2000 Jul;41(7):287-91.

[7] Rostami M, Tateyama S, Uchida K, Naitou H, Yamaguchi R, Otsuka H (1994) Tumours in domestic animals examined during a ten-year period (1980 to 1989) at Miyazaki University. *J. Vet. Med. Sci.* 56, 403-405.

[8] Johnston SD (1993) Reproductive systems. In Slatter (ed.): *Textbook of Small Animal Surgery,* 2nd ed., vol.2, W B Saunders, Philadelphia,

[9] Gobello C, Corrada Y (2001) Canine Mammary Tumors: An Endocrine Clinical Approach. *Compend. Contin. Educ. Pract. Vet.* 23, 705-709.

[10] Ferguson HR. Canine mammary gland tumors. *Vet. Clin. North Am. Small Anim. Pract.* 1985 May;15(3):501-11.

[11] MacVean DW, Monlux AW, Anderson PS Jr, Silberg SL, Roszel JF. Frequency of canine and feline tumors in a defined population. *Vet. Pathol. 1*978 Nov;15(6):700-15.

[12] Sorenmo K. Canine mammary gland tumors. *Vet. Clin. North Am. Small Anim. Pract.* 2003 May;33(3):573-96.

[13] Antuofermo E, Miller MA, Pirino S, Xie J, Badve S, Mohammed SI.Spontaneous mammary intraepithelial lesions in dogs--a model of breast cancer. *Cancer Epidemiol Biomarkers Prev.* 2007 Nov;16(11):2247-56. Epub 2007 Nov 2.

[14] Mouser P, Miller MA, Antuofermo E, Badve SS, Mohammed SI. Prevalence and classification of spontaneous mammary intraepithelial lesions in dogs without clinical mammary disease. *Vet Pathol.* 2010 Mar;47(2):275-84. Epub 2010 Jan 22.

[15] Rutteman GR.Hormones and mammary tumour disease in the female dog: an update. *In Vivo*. 1990 Jan-Feb;4(1):33-40.

[16] Veronesi MC, Battocchio M, Rizzi C, Sironi G. Relationship between dysplastic and neoplastic mammary lesions and pseudopregnancy in the bitch. *Vet Res. Commun*. 2003 Sep;27 Suppl 1:245-7.

[17] Benjamin SA, Lee AC, Saunders WJ. Classification and behavior of canine mammary epithelial neoplasms based on life-span observations in beagles. *Vet Pathol*. 1999 Sep;36(5):423-36.

[18] Taylor GN, Shabestari L, Williams J, Mays CW, Angus W, McFarland S. Mammary neoplasia in a closed beagle colony. *Cancer Res*. 1976 Aug;36(8):2740-3.

[19] Schneider R, Dorn CR, Taylor DO. Factors influencing canine mammary cancer development and postsurgical survival. *J. Natl. Cancer Inst*. 1969 Dec;43(6):1249-61.

[20] Støvring M, Moe L, Glattre E.A population-based case-control study of canine mammary tumours and clinical use of medroxyprogesterone acetate. *APMIS*. 1997 Aug;105(8):590-6.

[21] Rutteman GR. Contraceptive steroids and the mammary gland: is there a hazard?--Insights from animal studies. Breast Cancer Res Treat. 1992;23(1-2):29-41.

[22] Sonnenschein EG, Glickman LT, Goldschmidt MH, McKee LJ.Body conformation, diet, and risk of breast cancer in pet dogs: a case-control study.*Am. J. Epidemiol*. 1991 Apr 1;133(7):694-703.

[23] Shofer FS, Sonnenshein EG, Goldschmidt MH, Laster LL, Glickman LT (1989) Histopathologic and dietary prognostic factors for canine mammary carcinoma. *Breast cancer Res. Treat*. 13, 49-60.

[24] Pérez Alenza D, Rutteman GR, Peña L, Beynen AC, Cuesta P. Relation between habitual diet and canine mammary tumors in a case-control study. *J. Vet Intern. Med*. 1998 May-Jun;12(3):132-9.

[25] King MC, Marks JH, Mandell JB; New York Breast Cancer Study Group.Breast and ovarian cancer risks due to inherited mutations in BRCA1 and BRCA2. *Science*. 2003 Oct 24;302(5645):643-6.

[26] Eisen A, Lubinski J, Klijn J, Moller P, Lynch HT, Offit K, Weber B, Rebbeck T, Neuhausen SL, Ghadirian P, Foulkes WD, Gershoni-Baruch R, Friedman E, Rennert G, Wagner T, Isaacs C, Kim-Sing C, Ainsworth P, Sun P, Narod SA.Breast cancer risk following bilateral oophorectomy in BRCA1 and BRCA2 mutation carriers: an international case-control study.*J. Clin. Oncol.* 2005 Oct 20;23(30):7491-6.

[27] Rivera P, Melin M, Biagi T, Fall T, Häggström J, Lindblad-Toh K, von Euler H.Mammary tumor development in dogs is associated with BRCA1 and BRCA2. *Cancer Res.* 2009 Nov 15;69(22):8770-4.

[28] Dias Pereira P, Lopes CC, Matos AJ, Pinto D, Gärtner F, Lopes C, Medeiros R. Estrogens metabolism associated with polymorphisms: influence of COMT G482a genotype on age at onset of canine mammary tumors.*Vet Pathol.* 2008 Mar;45(2):124-30.

[29] Madewell BR, Theilen GH: (1987) Tumors of the Mammary Gland. In Theilen GH, Madewell BR (eds): *Veterinary Cancer Medicine*, 2nd ed., Lea and Febiger, Philadelphia, pp. 327-344.

[30] Rutteman GR (1995) Mammary tumors in the dog. In Bonagura JD (ed.): Kirk's Current Veterinary *Therapy XII Small Animal Practice*, W. B. Saunders, Philadelphia, pp. 518-523.

[31] Sorenmo KU, Kristiansen VM, Cofone MA, Shofer FS, Breen AM, Langeland M, Mongil CM, Grondahl AM, Teige J, Goldschmidt MH. Canine mammary gland tumours; a histological continuum from benign to malignant; clinical and histopathological evidence. *Vet Comp. Oncol.* 2009 Sep;7(3):162-72.

[32] Rutteman GR, Misdorp W, Blankenstein MA, van den Brom WE. Oestrogen (ER) and progestin receptors (PR) in mammary tissue of the female dog: different receptor profile in non-malignant and malignant states. *Br. J. Cancer.* 1988 Nov;58(5):594-9.

[33] Gama A, Alves A, Schmitt F. Identification of molecular phenotypes in canine mammary carcinomas with clinical implications: application of the human classification. *Virchows Arch.* 2008 Aug;453(2):123-32.

[34] Chang CC, Tsai MH, Liao JW, Chan JP, Wong ML, Chang SC.Evaluation of hormone receptor expression for use in predicting survival of female dogs with malignant mammary gland tumors. *J. Am. Vet Med. Assoc.* 2009 Aug 15;235(4):391-6.

[35] Misdorp W, 2002: Tumours of the mammary gland. In: Meuten DJ (ed.), *Tumours in Domestic Animals,* 4th edn Iowa State Press, Ames, 575-606.

[36] Rutteman GR, Cornelisse CJ, Dijkshoorn NJ, Poortman J, Misdorp W. Flow cytometric analysis of DNA ploidy in canine mammary tumors. Cancer Res. 1988 Jun 15;48(12):3411-7.

[37] Sautet JY, Ruberte J, Lopez C. Lymphatic system of the mammary glands in the dog: an approach to the surgical treatment of malignant mammary tumors. Canine Pract. 1992; 17: 30-33.

[38] Silver IA.The anatomy of the mammary gland of the dog and cat. *J. Small Anim. Pract.* 1966 Nov;7(11):689-96.

[39] Pereira CT, Rahal SC, de Carvalho Balieiro JC, Ribeiro AA.Lymphatic drainage on healthy and neoplasic mammary glands in female dogs: can it really be altered? *Anat. Histol. Embryol.* 2003 Oct;32(5):282-90.

[40] Chambers AF, Groom AC, MacDonald IC. Dissemination and growth of cancer cells in metastatic sites. *Nat. Rev. Cancer.* 2002 Aug;2(8):563-72.

[41] Sporn MB. The war on cancer. *Lancet.* 1996 May 18;347(9012): 1377-81.

[42] Kopfstein L, Christofori G. Metastasis: cell-autonomous mechanisms versus contributions by the tumor microenvironment. *Cell Mol. Life Sci.* 2006 Feb;63(4):449-68.

[43] de Oliveira JT, de Matos AJ, Gomes J, Vilanova M, Hespanhol V, Manninen A, Rutteman G, Chammas R, Gärtner F, Bernardes ES.Coordinated expression of galectin-3 and galectin-3-binding sites in malignant mammary tumors: implications for tumor metastasis. *Glycobiology.* 2010 Nov;20(11):1341-52.

[44] de Oliveira JT, de Matos AJ, Santos AL, Pinto R, Gomes J, Hespanhol V, Chammas R, Manninen A, Bernardes ES, Albuquerque Reis C, Rutteman G, Gärtner F. Sialylation regulates galectin-3/ligand interplay during mammary tumour progression - a case of targeted uncloaking. *Int. J. Dev. Biol.* 2011;55(7-8-9):823-834.

[45] de Oliveira JT, de Matos AJ, Barros R, Chen A, Hespanhol V, Rutteman G, Gärtner F. *Differential expression of galectin-1 and galectin-3 in mammary tumours: complementary roles in progression and invasion.* (In preparation).

[46] Cassali GD, Gobbi H, Malm C, Schmitt FC.Evaluation of accuracy of fine needle aspiration cytology for diagnosis of canine mammary tumours: comparative features with human tumours. *Cytopathology.* 2007 Jun;18(3):191-6.

[47] Simon D, Schoenrock D, Nolte I, Baumgärtner W, Barron R, Mischke R. Cytologic examination of fine-needle aspirates from mammary gland tumors in the dog: diagnostic accuracy with comparison to histopathology and association with postoperative outcome. *Vet Clin. Pathol.* 2009 Dec;38(4):521-8.

[48] Fossum TW, Hedlund CS, 1997: Mammary neoplasia. In: Duncan L (ed.), *Small Animal Surgery.* Don. Ladig, St. Louis 539-544.

[49] Nemanic S, London CA, Wisner ER. Comparison of thoracic radiographs and single breath-hold helical CT for detection of pulmonary nodules in dogs with metastatic neoplasia. *J. Vet Intern. Med.* 2006 May-Jun;20(3):508-15.

[50] Misdorp W, Else RW, Hellmén E, Lipscomb TP (1999) Histological Classification of Mammary Tumors of the Dog and the Cat. *World Health Organization Histological Classification of Tumors of Domestic Animals,* second series, vol. 7, n 2. Armed Forces Institute of Pathology, Washington, D.C.

[51] Elston CW, Ellis IO.Pathological prognostic factors in breast cancer. I. The value of histological grade in breast cancer: experience from a large study with long-term follow-up. C. W. Elston and I. O. Ellis. Histopathology 1991; 19; 403-410. *Histopathology.* 2002 Sep;41 (3A):151-2, discussion 152-3.

[52] de Oliveira JT, Pinho SS, de Matos AJ, Hespanhol V, Reis CA, Gärtner F. MUC1 expression in canine malignant mammary tumours and relationship to clinicopathological features. *Vet J.* 2009 Dec;182(3): 491-3.

[53] Santos AA, Oliveira JT, Lopes CC, Amorim IF, Vicente CM, Gärtner FR, Matos AJ. Immunohistochemical expression of vascular endothelial growth factor in canine mammary tumours. *J. Comp. Pathol.* 2010 Nov;143(4):268-75. Epub 2010 Jun 8.

[54] Sassi F, Benazzi C, Castellani G, Sarli G. Molecular-based tumour subtypes of canine mammary carcinomas assessed by immunohistochemistry. *BMC Vet Res.* 2010 Jan 28;6:5.

[55] Matos AJ, Faustino AM, Lopes C, Rutteman GR, Gärtner F. Detection of lymph node micrometastases in malignant mammary tumours in dogs by cytokeratin immunostaining. *Vet Rec.* 2006 May 6;158(18):626-30.

[56] Stratmann N, Failing K, Richter A, Wehrend A.Mammary tumor recurrence in bitches after regional mastectomy. *Vet Surg.* 2008 Jan;37(1):82-6.

[57] Clifford EJ, De Vol EB, Pockaj BA, Wilke LG, Boughey JC. Early results from a novel quality outcomes program: the American Society Of Breast Surgeons' Mastery of Breast Surgery. *Ann. Surg. Oncol.* 2010 Oct;17 Suppl 3:233-41.

[58] Jahanzeb M. Reducing the risk for breast cancer recurrence after completion of tamoxifen treatment in postmenopausal women. Clin Ther. 2007 Aug;29(8):1535-47.

[59] Marconato L, Lorenzo R, Abramo F, Ratto A, Zini E (2008) Adjuvant gemcitabine after surgical removal of aggressive malignant mammary tumours in dogs. *Veterinary and Comparative Oncology* 6, 90-101.

[60] Yamashita A, Maruo K, Suzuki K, Shirota K, Kobayashi K, Hioki K (2001) Experimental chemotherapy against canine mammary cancer xenograft in SCID mice and its prediction of clinical effect. *Journal of Veterinary Medical Sciences* 63, 831-836.

[61] Karayannopoulou M, Kaldrymidou E, Constantinidis T, Dessiris A (2001) Adjuvant post-operative chemotherapy in bitches with mammary cancer. *Journal of Veterinary Medical Association* 48, 85-96.

[62] Silver DP, Richardson AL, Eklund AC, Wang ZC, Szallasi Z, Li Q, Juul N, Leong CO, Calogrias D, Buraimoh A, Fatima A, Gelman RS, Ryan PD, Tung NM, De Nicolo A, Ganesan S, Miron A, Colin C, Sgroi DC, Ellisen LW, Winer EP, Garber JE. Efficacy of neoadjuvant Cisplatin in triple-negative breast cancer. *J. Clin. Oncol.* 2010 Mar 1;28(7):1145-53.

[63] Ellis P, Barrett-Lee P, Johnson L, Cameron D, Wardley A, O'Reilly S, Verrill M, Smith I, Yarnold J, Coleman R, Earl H, Canney P, Twelves C, Poole C, Bloomfield D, Hopwood P, Johnston S, Dowsett M, Bartlett JM, Ellis I, Peckitt C, Hall E, Bliss JM; TACT Trial Management Group; TACT Trialists. Sequential docetaxel as adjuvant chemotherapy for early breast cancer (TACT): an open-label, phase III, randomised controlled trial. *Lancet.* 2009 May 16;373(9676):1681-92.

[64] Burnell M, Levine MN, Chapman JA, Bramwell V, Gelmon K, Walley B, Vandenberg T, Chalchal H, Albain KS, Perez EA, Rugo H, Pritchard K, O'Brien P, Shepherd LE. Cyclophosphamide, epirubicin, and Fluorouracil versus dose-dense epirubicin and cyclophosphamide followed by Paclitaxel versus Doxorubicin and cyclophosphamide followed by Paclitaxel in node-positive or high-risk node-negative breast cancer.*J. Clin. Oncol.* 2010 Jan 1;28(1):77-82.

[65] McEntee M, Rassnick K, Lewis L, Zgola M, Beaulieu B, Balkman C, Page R (2006) Phase I and pharmacokinetic evaluation of the combination of orally administered docetaxel and cyclosporin A in tumour-bearing dogs. *American Journal of Veterinary Research* 67, 1057-1062.

[66] Poirier V, Hershey A, Burgess K, Philips B, Turek M, Forrest L, Beaver L, Vail D (2004) Efficacy and toxicity of paclitaxel (taxol) for the treatment of canine malignant tumours. *Journal of Veterinary Internal Medicine* 18, 219-222.

[67] Simon D, Schoenrock D, Baumgärtner W, Nolte I (2006) Postoperative adjuvant treatment of invasive malignant mammary gland tumours in dogs with doxorrubicin and docetaxel. *Journal of Veterinary Internal Medicine* 20, 1184-1190.

[68] Knoop AS, Knudsen H, Balslev E, Rasmussen BB, Overgaard J, Nielsen KV, Schonau A, Gunnarsdóttir K, Olsen KE, Mouridsen H, Ejlertsen B; Danish Breast Cancer Cooperative Group.retrospective analysis of topoisomerase IIa amplifications and deletions as predictive markers in primary breast cancer patients randomly assigned to cyclophosphamide, methotrexate, and fluorouracil or cyclophosphamide, epirubicin, and fluorouracil: Danish Breast Cancer Cooperative Group. *J. Clin. Oncol.* 2005 Oct 20;23(30):7483-90.

[69] Shenkier T, Weir L, Levine M, Olivotto I, Whelan T, Reyno L; Steering Committee on Clinical Practice Guidelines for the Care and Treatment of Breast Cancer. Clinical practice guidelines for the care and treatment of breast cancer: 15. Treatment for women with stage III or locally advanced breast cancer. *CMAJ.* 2004 Mar 16;170(6):983-94.

[70] Nowak M, Madej JA, Dziegiel P. Expression of Breast Cancer Resistance Protein (BCRP-1) in canine mammary adenocarcinomas and adenomas. In Vivo. 2009 Sep-Oct;23(5):705-9.

[71] Martelli G, DePalo G, Rossi N, Coradini D, Boracchi P, Galante E, Vetrella G. Long-term follow-up of elderly patients with operable breast cancer treated with surgery without axillary dissection plus adjuvant tamoxifen. *Br. J. Cancer.* 1995 Nov;72(5):1251-5.

[72] Sartin E, Barnes S, Toivio-Kinnucan M, Wright J, Wolfe L (1993) Heterogenic properties of clonal cell lines derived from canine mammary carcinomas and sensitivity to tamoxifen and doxorubicin. *Anticancer Research* 13, 229-236.

[73] Morris J, Dobson J, Bostock D (1993) Use of tamoxifen in the control of canine mammary neoplasia. *Veterinary Record* 27, 539-542.

[74] Yamagami T, Kobayashi T, Takahashi K, Sugiyama M (1996) Influence of ovariectomy on the prognosis for canine malignant mammary tumours. *Journal of small animal practice* 37, 462-464.

[75] Morris J, Dobson J, Bostock D, O'Farrell E (1998) Effect of ovariohysterectomy in bitches with mammary neoplasms. *Veterinary Record* 142, 656-658.

[76] Sorenmo KU, Shofer FS, Goldschmidt MH. Effect of spaying and timing of spaying on survival of dogs with mammary carcinoma. *J. Vet. Intern. Med.* 2000 May-Jun;14(3):266-70.

[77] Philibert JC, Snyder PW, Glickman N, Glickman LT, Knapp DW, Waters DJ. Influence of host factors on survival in dogs with malignant mammary gland tumors. *J. Vet. Intern. Med.* 2003 Jan-Feb;17(1):102-6.

[78] Guil-Luna S, Sánchez-Céspedes R, Millán Y, De Andrés FJ, Rollón E, Domingo V, Guscetti F, Martín de Las Mulas J. Aglepristone decreases proliferation in progesterone receptor-positive canine mammary carcinomas. *J. Vet. Intern. Med.* 2011 May-Jun;25(3):518-23.

[79] Lombardi P, Florio S, Pagnini U, Crispino A, Avallone L. Ovarian function suppression with a GnRH analogue: D-ser(But[t])[6]-Arzgly[10]-LHRH (Goserelin) in hormone dependent canine mammary cancer. *J. Vet. Pharmacol. Ther.* 1999 Feb;22(1):56-61.

[80] Hermo GA, Torres P, Ripoll GV, Scursoni AM, Gomez DE, Alonso DF, Gobello C. Perioperative desmopressin prolongs survival in surgically treated bitches with mammary gland tumours: a pilot study. *Vet. J.* 2008 Oct;178(1):103-8.

[81] Hermo GA, Turic E, Angelico D, Scursoni AM, Gomez DE, Gobello C, Alonso DF. Effect of adjuvant perioperative desmopressin in locally advanced canine mammary carcinoma and its relation to histologic grade. *J. Am. Anim. Hosp. Assoc.* 2011 Jan-Feb;47(1):21-7.

[82] Poirier VJ, Burgess KE, Adams WM, Vail DM.Toxicity, dosage, and efficacy of vinorelbine (Navelbine) in dogs with spontaneous neoplasia. *J. Vet. Intern. Med.* 2004 Jul-Aug;18(4):536-9.

[83] Grant IA, Rodriguez CO, Kent MS, Sfilgoi G, Gordon I, Davis G, Lord L, London CA. A phase II clinical trial of vinorelbine in dogs with cutaneous mast cell tumors. *J. Vet. Intern. Med.* 2008 Mar-Apr;22(2):388-93.

[84] Coleman RE, Marshall H, Cameron D, Dodwell D, Burkinshaw R, Keane M, Gil M, Houston SJ, Grieve RJ, Barrett-Lee PJ, Ritchie D, Pugh J, Gaunt C, Rea U, Peterson J, Davies C, Hiley V, Gregory W, Bell R; AZURE investigators.Breast-cancer adjuvant therapy with zoledronic acid. *N. Engl. J. Med.* 2011 Oct 13;365(15):1396-405.

[85] Spugnini EP, Vincenzi B, Caruso G, Baldi A, Citro G, Santini D, Tonini G. Zoledronic acid for the treatment of appendicular osteosarcoma in a dog. *J. Small Anim. Pract.* 2009 Jan;50(1):44-6.

[86] Peña LL, Nieto AI, Pérez-Alenza D, Cuesta P, Castaño M (1998) Immunohistochemical detection of Ki-67 and PCNA in canine mammary tumors: relationship to clinical and pathologic variables. *J. Vet. Diagn. Invest.* 10, 237-246.

[87] Chang SC, Chang CC, Chang TJ, Wong ML (2005) Prognostic factors associated withsurvival two years after surgery in dogs with malignant mammary tumours: 79 cases (1998-2002). *J. Am. Vet. Med. Ass.* 227, 1625-1629.

[88] De las Mulas J, Millán Y, Dios R (2005) A prospective analysis of immunohistochemically determined estrogen receptor □and progesterone receptor expression and host and tumour factors as predictors of disease-free period in mammary tumours of the dog. *Vet. Pathol.* 42, 200-212.

[89] Hellmén E, Bergström R, Holmberg L, Spångberg I-B, Hansson K, Lindgren A (1993) Prognostic factors in canine mammary tumors: A multivariate study of 202 consecutivecases. *Vet. Pathol.* 30, 20-27.

[90] Pérez-Alenza MD, Peña L, Nieto AI, Castaño M (1997) Clinical and pathologicalprognostic factors in canine mammary tumors. *Ann. Inst. Super. Sanità* 33, 581-585.

[91] Misdorp W, Hart AA (1976) Prognostic factors in canine mammary cancer. *J. Natl. Cancer Inst.* 56, 779- 786.

[92] Sarli G, Preziozi R, Benazzi C, Castellani G, Marcato PS (2002) Prognostic value of histologic stage and proliferative activity in canie malignant mammary tumors. *J. Vet. Diagn. Invest.* 14, 25-34.

[93] Karayannopoulou M, Kaldrymidou E, Constantinidis TC, Dessiris A. Histological grading and prognosis in dogs with mammary carcinomas: application of a human grading method. *J. Comp. Pathol.* 2005 Nov;133(4):246-52.

[94] Rutteman GR, Misdorp W (1993) Hormonal background of canine and feline mammary tumours. *J. Reprod Fertil. Suppl.* 47, 483-487.

[95] da Costa A, Oliveira JT, Gärtner F, Kohn B, Gruber AD, Klopfleisch R. Potential markers for detection of circulating canine mammary tumor cells in the peripheral blood. *Vet J.* 2011 Oct;190(1):165-8.

[96] Lee CH, Kweon OK. Mutations of p53 tumor suppressor gene in spontaneous canine mammary tumors. *J. Vet Sci.* 2002 Dec;3(4):321-5.

[97] Dias Pereira P, Lopes CC, Matos AJ, Pinto D, Gärtner F, Lopes C, Medeiros R. Influence of catechol-O-methyltransferase (COMT) genotypes on the prognosis of canine mammary tumors. *Vet Pathol.* 2009 Nov;46(6):1270-4.

[98] Nieto AI, Peña L, Pérez-Alenza MD, Sánchez MA, Flores JM, Castaño M (2000) Immunohistologic detection of estrogen receptor alpha in canine mammary tumors: clinical and pathologic associations and prognostic significance. *Vet Pathol.* 37, 239-247.

[99] Pereira PD, Lopes CC, Matos AJ, Cortez PP, Gärtner F, Medeiros R, Lopes C. Caveolin-1 in diagnosis and prognosis of canine mammary tumours: comparison of evaluation systems. *J. Comp. Pathol.* 2010 Aug-Oct;143(2-3):87-93.

[100] Lavalle GE, Bertagnolli AC, Tavares WL, Cassali GD.Cox-2 expression in canine mammary carcinomas: correlation with angiogenesis and overall survival. *Vet Pathol.* 2009 Nov;46(6):1275-80.

[101] Gama A, Paredes J, Gärtner F, Alves A, Schmitt F. Expression of E-cadherin, P-cadherin and beta-catenin in canine malignant mammary

tumours in relation to clinicopathological parameters, proliferation and survival. *Vet J.* 2008 Jul;177(1):45-53.

[102] Matos AJ, Lopes C, Carvalheira J, Santos M, Rutteman GR, Gärtner F. E-cadherin expression in canine malignant mammary tumours: relationship to other clinico-pathological variables. *J. Comp. Pathol.* 2006 Feb-Apr;134(2-3):182-9.

[103] Santos A, Lopes C, Frias C, Amorim I, Vicente C, Gärtner F, Matos A. Immunohistochemical evaluation of MMP-2 and TIMP-2 in canine mammary tumours: A survival study. *Vet J.* 2011 Dec;190(3):396-402.

[104] Santos A, Lopes C, Marques RM, Amorim I, Ribeiro J, Frias C, Vicente C, Gärtner F, de Matos A. Immunohistochemical analysis of urokinase plasminogen activator and its prognostic value in canine mammary tumours. *Vet J.* 2011 Jul;189(1):43-8.

[105] Liu FT, Rabinovich GA.Galectins as modulators of tumour progression. *Nat. Rev. Cancer.* 2005 Jan;5(1):29-41.

[106] Puche AC, Poirier F, Hair M, Bartlett PF, Key B. Role of galectin-1 in the developing mouse olfactory system. *Dev. Biol.* 1996 Oct 10;179(1):274-87.

[107] Colnot C, Ripoche MA, Milon G, Montagutelli X, Crocker PR, Poirier F. Maintenance of granulocyte numbers during acute peritonitis is defective in galectin-3-null mutant mice. *Immunology.* 1998 Jul;94(3):290-6.

[108] Sörme, P., Kahl-Knutsson, B., Wellmar, U., Magnusson, B. G., Leffler, H., Nilsson, U. J. (2003) Design and synthesis of galectin inhibitors in Recognition of carbohydrates in biological systems, part B: specific applications. *Meth. Enzymol.* 363,157-169.

[109] Seetharaman, J., Kanigsberg, A., Slaaby, R., Leffler, H., Barondes, S. H., Rini, J. M. (1998) X-ray crystal structure of the human galectin-3 carbohydrate recognition domain at 2.1-angstrom resolution. *J. Biol. Chem.* 273,13047-13052.

[110] Collins, P., Hidari, K. I. P. J., Blanchard, H. (2007) Slow diffusion of lactose out of galectin-3 crystals monitored by X-ray crystallography: possible implications for ligand-exchange protocols. *Acta Crystallogr.* D63,415-419.

[111] Sörme, P., Arnoux, P., Kahl-Knutsson, B., Leffler, H., Rini, J. M., Nilsson, L. J. (2005) Structural and thermodynamic studies on cation-II interactions in lectin-ligand complexes: high-affinity galectin-3

inhibitors through fine-tuning of an arginine-arene interaction. *J. Am. Chem. Soc.* 127,1737-1743.

[112] Sathisha, U. V., Jayaram, S., Hayaka, M. A. H., Dharmash, S. M. (2007) Inhibition of galectin-3 mediated cellular interactions by pectic polysaccharides from dietary sources. *Glycoconj. J.* 24,497-507.

[113] Beuth, J., Ko, H. L., Schirrmacher, V., Uhlenbruck, G., Pulverer, G. (1988) Inhibition of liver-tumor cell colonisation in 2 animal tumor-models by lectin blocking with D-galactose or arabinogalactan. *Clin. Exper. Metastasis* 6,115-120.

[114] Uhlenbruk, G., Beuth, J., Oette, K., Roszkowski, W., Ko, H. L., Pulverer, G. (1986) Prevention of experimental liver metastasis by arabinogalactan. *Naturwissenschaften* 73,626-627.

[115] Vayssade M, Sengkhamparn N, Verhoef R, Delaigue C, Goundiam O, Vigneron P, Voragen AG, Schols HA, Nagel MD. Antiproliferative and proapoptotic actions of okra pectin on B16F10 melanoma cells. *Phytother Res.* 2010 Jul;24(7):982-9.

[116] Sörme, P., Kahl-Knutsson, B., Carlsson, S., Nilsson, U. J., Arnoux, P., Rini, J. M., Leffler, H. (2003) The design of monovalent galectin inhibitors based on 3-OH-modified galactosides. *FASEB J.* 17, A162-A162.

[117] Glinsky VV, Kiriakova G, Glinskii OV, Mossine VV, Mawhinney TP, Turk JR, Glinskii AB, Huxley VH, Price JE, Glinsky GV. Synthetic galectin-3 inhibitor increases metastatic cancer cell sensitivity to taxol-induced apoptosis in vitro and in vivo. *Neoplasia.* 2009 Sep;11(9):901-9.

[118] Arnusch CJ, André S, Valentini P, Lensch M, Russwurm R, Siebert HC, Fischer MJ, Gabius HJ, Pieters RJ. Interference of the galactose-dependent binding of lectins by novel pentapeptide ligands. *Bioorg. Med. Chem. Lett.* 2004 Mar 22;14(6):1437-40.

[119] Pieters RJ. Inhibition and detection of galectins. *Chembiochem.* 2006 May;7(5):721-8.

[120] Dunn GP, Old LJ, Schreiber RD. The immunobiology of cancer immunosurveillance and immunoediting. *Immunity.* 2004 Aug;21(2): 137-48.

[121] Lin EY, Pollard JW. Role of infiltrated leucocytes in tumour growth and spread. *Br. J. Cancer.* 2004 Jun 1;90(11):2053-8.

[122] Rabinovich GA, Baum LG, Tinari N, Paganelli R, Natoli C, Liu FT, Iacobelli S. Galectins and their ligands: amplifiers, silencers or tuners of the inflammatory response? *Trends Immunol.* 2002 Jun;23(6):313-20.

[123] He J, Baum LG. Presentation of galectin-1 by extracellular matrix triggers T cell death. *J. Biol. Chem.* 2004 Feb 6;279(6):4705-12.

[124] Rubinstein N, Alvarez M, Zwirner NW, Toscano MA, Ilarregui JM, Bravo A, Mordoh J, Fainboim L, Podhajcer OL, Rabinovich GA. Targeted inhibition of galectin-1 gene expression in tumor cells results in heightened T cell-mediated rejection; A potential mechanism of tumor-immune privilege. *Cancer Cell.* 2004 Mar;5(3):241-51.

[125] Yamaoka K, Mishima K, Nagashima Y, Asai A, Sanai Y, Kirino T. Expression of galectin-1 mRNA correlates with the malignant potential of human gliomas and expression of antisense galectin-1 inhibits the growth of 9 glioma cells. *J. Neurosci. Res.* 2000 Mar 15;59(6):722-30.

[126] Ingber DE. Extracellular matrix as a solid-state regulator in angiogenesis: identification of new targets for anti-cancer therapy. *Semin Cancer Biol.* 1992

[127] Carmeliet P, Dor Y, Herbert JM, Fukumura D, Brusselmans K, Dewerchin M, Neeman M, Bono F, Abramovitch R, Maxwell P, Koch CJ, Ratcliffe P, Moons L, Jain RK, Collen D, Keshert E. Role of HIF-1alpha in hypoxia-mediated apoptosis, cell proliferation and tumour angiogenesis. *Nature.* 1998 Jul 30;394(6692):485-90.

[128] Semenza GL. Hypoxia-inducible factor 1: master regulator of O2 homeostasis. *Curr. Opin. Genet. Dev.* 1998 Oct;8(5):588-94.

[129] Le Mercier M, Fortin S, Mathieu V, Kiss R, Lefranc F Galectins and gliomas. *Brain Pathol.* 2010 Jan;20(1):17-27.

[130] Markowska AI, Liu FT, Panjwani N. Galectin-3 is an important mediator of VEGF- and bFGF-mediated angiogenic response. *J. Exp. Med.* 2010 Aug 30;207(9):1981-93.

[131] Nangia-Makker P, Hogan V, Honjo Y, Baccarini S, Tait L, Bresalier R, Raz A. Inhibition of human cancer cell growth and metastasis in nude mice by oral intake of modified citrus pectin. *J. Natl. Cancer Inst.* 2002 Dec 18;94(24):1854-62.

[132] Nangia-Makker P, Honjo Y, Sarvis R, Akahani S, Hogan V, Pienta KJ, Raz A. Galectin-3 induces endothelial cell morphogenesis and angiogenesis. *Am. J. Pathol.* 2000 Mar;156(3):899-909.

[133] Kim HR, Lin HM, Biliran H, Raz A. Cell cycle arrest and inhibition of anoikis by galectin-3 in human breast epithelial cells. *Cancer Res.* 1999 Aug 15;59(16):4148-54.

[134] Matarrese P, Tinari N, Semeraro ML, Natoli C, Iacobelli S, Malorni W. Galectin-3 overexpression protects from cell damage and death by influencing mitochondrial homeostasis. *FEBS Lett.* 2000 May 19;473(3): 311-5.

[135] Sanchez-Ruderisch H, Fischer C, Detjen KM, Welzel M, Wimmel A, Manning JC, André S, Gabius HJ.Tumor suppressor p16 INK4a: Downregulation of galectin-3, an endogenous competitor of the pro-anoikis effector galectin-1, in a pancreatic carcinoma model. *FEBS J.* 2010 Sep;277(17):3552-63.

[136] Zhao Q, Barclay M, Hilkens J, Guo X, Barrow H, Rhodes JM, Yu LG. Interaction between circulating galectin-3 and cancer-associated MUC1 enhances tumour cell homotypic aggregation and prevents anoikis. *Mol. Cancer.* 2010 Jun 18;9:154.

[137] Al-Mehdi AB, Tozawa K, Fisher AB, Shientag L, Lee A, Muschel RJ. Intravascular origin of metastasis from the proliferation of endothelium-attached tumor cells: a new model for metastasis. *Nat. Med.* 2000 Jan;6(1):100-2.

[138] Lehr JE, Pienta KJ. Preferential adhesion of prostate cancer cells to a human bone marrow endothelial cell line. *J. Natl. Cancer Inst.* 1998 Jan 21;90(2):118-23.

[139] Glinsky VV, Glinsky GV, Rittenhouse-Olson K, Huflejt ME, Glinskii OV, Deutscher SL, Quinn TP. The role of Thomsen-Friedenreich antigen in adhesion of human breast and prostate cancer cells to the endothelium. *Cancer Res.* 2001 Jun 15;61(12):4851-7.

[140] Glinsky VV, Glinsky GV, Glinskii OV, Huxley VH, Turk JR, Mossine VV, Deutscher SL, Pienta KJ, Quinn TP. Intravascular metastatic cancer cell homotypic aggregation at the sites of primary attachment to the endothelium. *Cancer Res.* 2003 Jul 1;63(13):3805-11.

[141] Khaldoyanidi SK, Glinsky VV, Sikora L, Glinskii AB, Mossine VV, Quinn TP, Glinsky GV, Sriramarao P. MDA-MB-435 human breast carcinoma cell homo- and heterotypic adhesion under flow conditions is mediated in part by Thomsen-Friedenreich antigen-galectin-3 interactions. *J. Biol. Chem.* 2003 Feb 7;278(6):4127-34.

[142] Platt D, Raz A. Modulation of the lung colonization of B16-F1 melanoma cells by citrus pectin. *J. Natl. Cancer Inst.* 1992 Mar 18;84(6):438-42.

[143] Pienta KJ, Naik H, Akhtar A, Yamazaki K, Replogle TS, Lehr J, Donat TL, Tait L, Hogan V, Raz A.Inhibition of spontaneous metastasis in a rat prostate cancer model by oral administration of modified citrus pectin. *J. Natl. Cancer Inst.* 1995 Mar 1;87(5):348-53.

[144] Inohara H, Raz A. Effects of natural complex carbohydrate (citrus pectin) on murine melanoma cell properties related to galectin-3 functions. *Glycoconj J.* 1994 Dec;11(6):527-32.

[145] van den Brûle FA, Buicu C, Baldet M, Sobel ME, Cooper DN, Marschal P, Castronovo V. Galectin-1 modulates human melanoma cell adhesion to laminin. *Biochem. Biophys. Res. Commun.* 1995 Apr 17;209(2):760-7.

[146] Ellerhorst J, Nguyen T, Cooper DN, Lotan D, Lotan R. Differential expression of endogenous galectin-1 and galectin-3 in human prostate cancer cell lines and effects of overexpressing galectin-1 on cell phenotype. *Int. J. Oncol.* 1999 Feb;14(2):217-24.

[147] Rorive S, Belot N, Decaestecker C, Lefranc F, Gordower L, Micik S, Maurage CA, Kaltner H, Ruchoux MM, Danguy A, Gabius HJ, Salmon I, Kiss R, Camby I. Galectin-1 is highly expressed in human gliomas with relevance for modulation of invasion of tumor astrocytes into the brain parenchyma. *Glia.* 2001 Mar 1;33(3):241-55. Erratum in: Glia 2001 Aug;35(2):166.

[148] Sathisha UV, Jayaram S, Harish Nayaka MA, Dharmesh SM. Inhibition of galectin-3 mediated cellular interactions by pectic polysaccharides from dietary sources. *Glycoconj J.* 2007 Nov;24(8): 497-507.

[149] Nangia-Makker P, Nakahara S, Hogan V, Raz A. Galectin-3 in apoptosis, a novel therapeutic target. *J. Bioenerg. Biomembr.* 2007 Feb;39(1):79-84.

[150] Califice S, Castronovo V, Bracke M, van den Brûle F. Dual activities of galectin-3 in human prostate cancer: tumor suppression of nuclear galectin-3 vs tumor promotion of cytoplasmic galectin-3. *Oncogene.* 2004 Sep 30;23(45):7527-36.

[151] Pommier Y, Sordet O, Antony S, Hayward RL, Kohn KW. Apoptosis defects and chemotherapy resistance: molecular interaction maps and networks. *Oncogene.* 2004 Apr 12;23(16):2934-49.

[152] Fukumori T, Oka N, Takenaka Y, Nangia-Makker P, Elsamman E, Kasai T, Shono M, Kanayama HO, Ellerhorst J, Lotan R, Raz A. Galectin-3 regulates mitochondrial stability and antiapoptotic function in response to anticancer drug in prostate cancer. *Cancer Res.* 2006 Mar 15;66(6):3114-9.

[153] Yu F, Finley RL Jr, Raz A, Kim HR. Galectin-3 translocates to the perinuclear membranes and inhibits cytochrome c release from the mitochondria. A role for synexin in galectin-3 translocation. *J. Biol. Chem.* 2002 May 3;277(18):15819-27.

[154] Fukumori T, Kanayama HO, Raz A.The role of galectin-3 in cancer drug resistance. *Drug Resist Updat.* 2007 Jun;10(3):101-8.

[155] Chauhan D, Li G, Podar K, Hideshima T, Neri P, He D, Mitsiades N, Richardson P, Chang Y, Schindler J, Carver B, Anderson KC. A novel carbohydrate-based therapeutic GCS-100 overcomes bortezomib resistance and enhances dexamethasone-induced apoptosis in multiple myeloma cells. *Cancer Res.* 2005 Sep 15;65(18):8350-8.

[156] Johnson KD, Glinskii OV, Mossine VV, Turk JR, Mawhinney TP, Anthony DC, Henry CJ, Huxley VH, Glinsky GV, Pienta KJ, Raz A, Glinsky VV. Galectin-3 as a potential therapeutic target in tumors arising from malignant endothelia. *Neoplasia.* 2007 Aug;9(8):662-70.

[157] Jackson CL, Dreaden TM, Theobald LK, Tran NM, Beal TL, Eid M, Gao MY, Shirley RB, Stoffel MT, Kumar MV, Mohnen D. Pectin induces apoptosis in human prostate cancer cells: correlation of apoptotic function with pectin structure. *Glycobiology.* 2007 Aug;17(8): 805-19.

[158] Hayashi A, Gillen AC, Lott JR. Effects of daily oral administration of quercetin chalcone and modified citrus pectin on implanted colon-25 tumor growth in Balb-c mice. *Altern. Med. Rev.* 2000 Dec;5(6):546-52.

[159] Gunning AP, Bongaerts RJ, Morris VJ. Recognition of galactan components of pectin by galectin-3. *FASEB J.* 2009 Feb;23(2):415-24.

[160] Guess BW, Scholz MC, Strum SB, Lam RY, Johnson HJ, Jennrich RI. Modified citrus pectin (MCP) increases the prostate-specific antigen doubling time in men with prostate cancer: a phase II pilot study. *Prostate Cancer Prostatic Dis.* 2003;6(4):301-4.

In: Canine Behavior, Classification and Diseases ISBN: 978-1-62081-304-1
Editors: R. L. Andrade and C. I. Batista

Chapter II

Gene Therapy for Canine Cancer: Clinical Results

Gerardo C. Glikin and Liliana M. E. Finocchiaro
Unidad de Transferencia Genética, Instituto de Oncología "Ángel H. Roffo", Universidad de Buenos Aires, Argentina

Abstract

Despite the important progress obtained in the treatment of some pets' malignancies, new treatments need to be developed. In this review we discuss the bases and we summarize the outcomes of published gene therapy veterinary clinical trials reported by many research centers up to date. A variety of tumors such as canine soft tissue sarcomas, osteosarcoma and lymphoma were subjected to different approaches. However, spontaneous canine melanoma (a highly aggressive tumor resistant to current therapies) was the preferred target. Both viral and mainly non-viral vectors as well as cytokine producing transgenic cells were used to deliver gene products as cytokines, suicide enzymes, xenogeneic tumor antigens, anti-angiogenic molecules and pro-apoptotic regulatory factors.

Among other examples, we are presenting our own successful experience with suicide plus immunogene therapy for spontaneous canine melanomas and sarcomas.

In general terms, very slight or no adverse collateral effects were found during this kind of treatments and usually treated patients displayed a better course of the disease (longer survival, delayed or suppressed local or systemic relapse, recovery of the quality of life), suggesting the utility of this sort of methodology as standard adjuvant treatment.

The encouraging outcomes obtained in companion animals support their ready application in veterinary clinical oncology and serve as preclinical proof of concept and safety assay for future human gene therapy trials.

Introduction

Gene therapy provides novel strategies to treat many cancers. The administration of a genetic vector can offer anti-tumor activity by converting transgenic cells into therapeutic protein factories *in situ*. Furthermore, direct gene transfer into the tumor may be able to restrict toxicity to localized areas while concentrating the therapeutic protein at the tumor site, without systemic toxicity. Besides targeting the tumor site for injection of vector, additional specificity can be obtained by using tumor-specific cell receptors and promoters, vectors that preferentially enter and express into tumor cells, and therapeutic genes that facilitate preferential killing of malignant cells.

Non-viral vectors offer an alternative to viral vectors for cancer gene therapy. Until recently non-viral vectors were limited by low gene transfer efficiency, rapidly declining gene expression, and poor distribution of gene transfer. Advances in physical and chemical methods to deliver plasmid DNA into tumor tissue and normal tissue are showing promise in narrowing the gap between viral and non-viral gene delivery efficiency [Ohlfest *et al.* 2005].

Amazingly cancer gene therapy clinical trials started much earlier in humans [Rosenberg *et al.*, 1990] than in companion animals [Quintin-Colonna *et al.*, 1996]. The convenience of a comparative oncology approach was extensively supported by Vail and MacEwen [2000] and Hansen and Khanna [2004], however there is a significantly higher number of human trials (1107 until June 2011, http://www.wiley.com/legacy/wileychi/genmed/clinical/).

Whereas nearly all the patients subjected to a variety of cancer gene therapy methodologies were canine, some data also raised from feline and equine patients [Finocchiaro and Glikin, 2008b]. As it is the case in human clinical trials, cancer immunogene therapy is largely leading the major attention. Different kinds of tumors were targeted, but spontaneous melanoma a highly aggressive tumor resistant to current therapies was the preferred model. Both viral and no-viral vectors as well as cytokine producing transgenic cells were used to deliver gene products as cytokines, suicide genes, tumor antigens and pro-apoptotic genes.

Even though large animals were involved in many gene therapy assays as reviewed by Casal *et al.* [2006], trials on spontaneous diseases were centered almost exclusively on cancer. We are currently focusing this review only on those papers reporting clinical data collected from client-owned patients with spontaneously arising tumors: those trials where the owners' informed written consent was granted and the welfare of the patients was a main concern. At present, an increasing number of non-invasive or slightly-invasive techniques that allow *in vivo* monitoring of treatments effects are available [Vassaux and Groot-Wassink, 2003] and they could be implemented soon to optimize the efficacy of the procedures.

The general trend in gene types used for canine cancer gene therapy clinical trials reflects what happens for humans, they were concentrated in three main gene types: 48% cytokines 32%, antigens, 12% suicide genes. Nevertheless, when vectors usage is analyzed, the pattern appears very different, most of trials used non-viral vectors: 36% lipofection, 24% naked plasmid electroporation, 12% naked plasmid jet injection and 8% gene gun. Merely 16% adenovirus and 4% retrovirus represented the viral vectors.

Canine Melanoma

The pioneering work of Quintin-Colonna *et al.* [1996] published about 15 years ago described an *ex vivo* genetically engineered xenogeneic cell gene therapy approach (that also could be defined as a transgenic xenogeneic cell therapy) for spontaneous canine melanoma. This highly aggressive tumor of the oral cavity, digit/footpad, and mucocutaneous junctions, appears clinically similar to aggressive human melanoma. Both diseases are chemo- and radio-resistant, do not respond well to treatment with conventional biological response modifiers and share similar metastatic phenotypes and site selectivity [Vail and MacEwen, 2000; Hansen and Khanna, 2004]. Like in human melanoma, the prognosis for canine melanoma correlates directly with tumor stage. At the time of diagnosis, the disease is often metastatic and has an extremely poor prognosis because rapid invasion of surrounding normal tissue and high likelihood of regional and distant metastasis early in the course of the disease. The high metastatic rate observed with this disease and the inefficacy of current therapies, warranted the investigation into novel therapies. In this work, the effects of repeated peritumoral local injections of human interleukin-2 (hIL-2) secreting Vero cells after surgical removal of the tumor followed by ^{60}Co-radiotherapy were evaluated. This combined treatment resulted in a considerably higher median survival of 270 days compared to 75 days of the surgery plus radiation controls (n=16, each group). The treatment resulted safe.

An individually targeted autologous *ex vivo* approach for spontaneous canine melanoma involving human granulocyte macrophage colony stimulating factor (hGM-CSF) gene transfer, was developed by Hogge *et al.* [1998]. In this case, after tumor removal, a suspension of tumor cells was subjected to a gene gun shot with gold particles coated with a plasmid carrying the human GM-CSF gene. After sub-lethal ^{137}Cs irradiation, transgenic cells were delivered as intra-dermal injections in the flank of the patients. As part of a phase I clinical trial, the treatment of 10 canine melanoma bearing patients resulted in 3 objective responses and 1 stable disease, while 3 cases of fibrosarcoma yielded 2 objective responses. No animal exhibited any signs of local or systemic toxicity. Even though statistically non significant because the low number of cases, survival time of melanoma responders (>300 days) largely exceeded the expected values for surgery treated patients (90-165 days).

By using intratumoral injections of bacterial superantigen gene (staphylococcal enterotoxin B, SEB) as immune-adjuvant plus immunostimulatory gene canine GM-CSF, Dow *et al.* [1998] informed the objective responses and median survivals for spontaneous canine melanoma as follows: stage I, 3/3-427 days; stage II, 3/5-399 days; stage III 4/12-168 days; stage IV, 0/2-n.d. Median survival (168 days) of stage III patients (n=12) resulted significantly higher than historical surgery controls (105 days). Intratumoral expression of SEB and canine GM-CSF genes carrying plasmid did not induce clinically important toxicity in treated dogs.

A totally different approach to promote immunologic "priming" through induction of apoptosis was assayed for canine melanoma by Bianco *et al.* [2003]. Direct intratumoral injections of a plasmid carrying the human Fas ligand (hFasL) gene caused a fast reduction (7 days) of tumor burden that was seen in 3 of 5 treated dogs. At that time, each dog was provided of standard care therapy as indicated for each tumor (surgery, radiation or palliation), and the final result was 4 objective responses with survivals ranging from 168 to 574 days. The treatment did not show any adverse effect.

On the other hand, Bergman *et al.* [2003] found that intramuscular needle free jet injection of a plasmid containing human tyrosinase gene and its expression as a melanoma xenoantigen considerably prolonged the median survival of canine melanoma bearing patients up to 389 days as compared with historical controls subjected to standard treatments (60-150 days). In addition, Liao *et al.* [2006] reported at least two long-term survivors displaying detectable levels of humoral anti-human tyrosinase antibodies. Fifty eight patients were enrolled in a larger trial to evaluate the safety and efficacy this DNA vaccine as adjunctive treatment for oral malignant canine melanoma in which locoregional disease control was achieved [Grosenbaugh *et al.*, 2011]. The median survival due to melanoma was significantly higher (>750 days) as compared to historical controls (324 days), and they reported only 14/58 deaths due to melanoma compared to 34/53 in historical controls reported by MacEwen *et al.* [1999]. They confirmed both safety and efficacy. As described by Bergman *et al.* [2006] other xenogeneic DNAs were assayed alone or combined, they coded for: murine tyrosinase, murine gp75 and human GM-CSF. Thirty-three stage II–III dogs with locoregionally controlled canine melanoma across the xenogeneic vaccine studies displayed a median survival time of 569 days, largely exceeding the value expected for standard treatments. Minimal to mild pain was noted at vaccination sites. All these results served to support the approval of the first therapeutic cancer vaccine available in the veterinary pharmaceutical market. As a continuation of these studies, Manley *et al.* [2011] determined the safety and effectiveness of the murine tyrosinase xenogeneic vaccine for canine digit melanoma when used in conjunction with local and regional disease control. This retrospective study suggests a prolongation of survival for dogs with melanoma of the digit treated with xenogeneic DNA melanoma vaccine (a median survival time: 476 days) compared with historical controls treated with surgery alone (a median survival time: 365 days). A survival advantage was noted for those dogs that were vaccinated near the time of diagnosis over those dogs that had a significant delay between diagnosis and vaccination.

Gyorffy *et al.* [2005] reported the feasibility of autologous dendritic cells pulsed with adenoviral vector encoding human gp100 applied as adjuvant of radiotherapy to treat canine melanoma. The 3 treated patients exceeded the expected median survival (210-1440 days), even though one died sooner because of progressive disease. No adverse effects were observed in any of the treated dogs with either the priming or the subsequent vaccine booster doses.

After vaccination with allogeneic cells expressing xenogeneic human gp100, Alexander *et al.* [2006] demonstrated that melanoma bearing dogs experiencing tumor control survived significantly longer than dogs having no response (median survivals: 337 days *vs.* 95 days). Adverse reactions were limited to mild induration and erythema at the site of vaccination.

A feasibility study was performed for adenovector CD40 ligand (CD40L) immunogene treatment [von Euler *et al.* 2008]. One case of advanced stage III oral melanoma, treated by intratumoral vaccination followed by cytoreductive surgery, did not relapse and survived 401 days. A second case of conjunctival malignant melanoma, treated only with intralesional injections, showed a continuous remission for more than 150 days. Only reversible minor side effects were reported.

By adding local *herpes simplex* virus thymidine kinase (HSV-*tk*) suicide gene bearing plasmid plus ganciclovir, in an approach that included intratumoral injections of xenogeneic hamster cells secreting hIL-2 and hGM-CSF (n=45), Finocchiaro *et al.* [2008] found that melanoma bearing dogs presenting local objective responses survived significantly longer than dogs lacking local objective responses (220 days *vs.* 151 days), being both responses considerably higher than those of surgery controls (82 days). As a continuation of these encouraging data, a surgery adjuvant treatment against the minimal residual disease whose rationale appeared to be considerably superior to the previous intratumoral treatment was assayed [Finocchiaro and Glikin, 2008a]. This new treatment consisted of complete or cytoreductive surgery followed by a combination of suicide gene therapy with a subcutaneous vaccine. This vaccine was a mixture of formolized tumor cells and irradiated xenogeneic cells producing hIL-2 and hGM-CSF. The post-surgical margin of the cavity was infiltrated with lipid-complexed HSV-*tk* suicide gene co-administrated with ganciclovir. Toxicity was minimal or absent in all patients. With respect to surgery treated controls, this combined treatment significantly increased the fraction of local disease-free patients from 6 to 58% and distant metastases-free patients from 43 to 78%. In addition, the combined treatment significantly improved both overall 78 (23-540) days and metastasis-free survival 112 (0-467) days of surgery treated controls to more than 1312 days (respective ranges: 43-1312 and 0-1312) (Kaplan-Meier analysis). In those patients subjected to partial surgery or presenting local recurrence, the efficacy of the local suicide gene approach was verified by a 49 % of objective responses that averaged 85% of tumor mass loss, while only 22% displayed tumor progression as 94% of the surgery controls did. This study suggested that the most optimal clinical setting is this surgery adjuvant treatment against minimal residual disease, a strong strategy that not only delays or prevents recurrence and distant metastasis, but substantially extends disease-free and overall survival, with a consequent improving in the quality of life.

Canine Soft Tissue Sarcoma

Soft-tissue sarcomas involve a group of tumors with differing morphological features that share similar biological behaviors. These tumors arise from many non-bony connective tissues and may originate in visceral and non-visceral sites, comprising approximately 15% of all skin and subcutaneous tumors in the dog [Ehrhart, 2005]. Wide surgical excision remains the cornerstone of treatment for these tumors. Local recurrence is common following conservative resection, and recurrent tumors are more difficult to treat.

A superantigen gene was assayed to enhance the action of immunostimulant cytokine gene, in this case against the invasive spontaneous canine soft tissue sarcoma that is refractory to most conventional therapies other than surgical excision. Thamm *et al.* [2003] reported the effects of intralesional treatment with a plasmid containing bacterial superantigen gene (staphylococcal enterotoxin A, SEA) plus immunostimulatory canine IL-2 gene before surgical resection or exploration and biopsy of the tumor bed. Median survival of the responders resulted >540 days without experiencing local recurrence or metastasis. Manageable transient adverse effects related to treatment were informed.

A polygene therapy approach was also assayed by Finocchiaro *et al.* [2011]. Eleven soft tissue sarcoma canine patients were subjected to: (i) periodic subcutaneous injection of irradiated xenogeneic cells secreting hGM-CSF and hIL-2 mixed with allogeneic or autologous tumor homogenates; and (ii) injections of cIFN-β and HSV-*tk*-carrying lipoplexes and ganciclovir, marginal (after surgery) and/or intratumoral (in the case of partial tumor resection, local relapse or small surface tumors). This treatment alone or as surgery adjuvant, was safe and well tolerated. In those patients presenting local disease (6/11), the suicide gene plus cIFN-β treatment induced local antitumor activity evidenced by the objective responses (3 complete, 1 partial) and stable diseases (2). In addition, the treatment prevented or delayed local relapse, regional metastases (lymph nodes developed only in 1/11) and distant metastases (0/11), suggesting a strong systemic antitumor immunity. Most of the patients displayed long survival times while maintaining a good quality of life: 2 about 4 years, 2 about 3 years, 1 more than 2 years, 4 more than 1 year, 2 more than 6 months).

Canine Osteosarcoma

Osteosarcoma accounts for approximately 85% of primary bone cancers in the dog [Mayer and Grier, 2006]. It is a common cancer of large to giant breed dogs, and it occurs primarily in the appendicular skeleton. Osteosarcoma in dogs is a common and highly metastatic tumor that biologically closely resembles osteosarcoma in humans [Vail and MacEwen, 2000; Hansen and Khanna, 2004], and does not have additional treatment options when adjuvant chemotherapy has failed against its disseminated form [Dow *et al.*, 2005]. Even with removal of the primary tumor before spread of the cancer is clinically detectable, metastases to lung, bone, or other sites eventually develop in almost all dogs [Mayer and Grier, 2006].

Metastatic disease often needs a systemic delivery of the therapeutic molecule to reach multiple points simultaneously. Systemic gene delivery by intravenous injection of cationic liposome-DNA complexes carrying canine IL-2 gene was assayed in 22 dogs with chemotherapy-resistant osteosarcoma lung metastases, as reported by Dow *et al.* [2005]. The treatment was well tolerated with 3 dogs displaying medium-term objective responses and 4 cases of stable disease. A significant increase of the median survival (82 d) with respect to untreated controls (58 d) was observed.

As it was the case for soft tissue sarcomas [Finocchiaro *et al.*, 2011], 6 osteosarcoma bearing patients were subjected to a treatment combining: (i) the local antiproliferative effects of interferon-β and HSV-*tk* suicide gene therapy with (ii) the systemic effects triggered by osteosarcoma antigens in an immunostimulatory environment created by the slow secretion of hGM-CSF and hIL-2 [Finocchiaro *et al.*, 2012]. Beyond the high safety standard of the proposed treatment on all the patients, 4 of them survived more than 6 months (among them, two exceeded 1 year). In addition, the treatment prevented or delayed local relapse, regional metastases and distant metastases, suggesting a strong systemic antitumor immunity. The use of this treatment after surgical removal of the tumor is safe and could delay or prevent post-surgical recurrence and metastases, with the consequent quality of life and survival rate improvement. In addition, when diagnosed at the early stages, a peritumoral application of interferon-β plus suicide genes in combination with subcutaneous vaccine could be effective in controlling both local (recurrence) and distant disease (metastases), as evidenced by one case of long-lasting complete remission (>453 days) without surgical intervention.

Canine Lymphoma

Canine lymphoma, one of the most common forms of cancer in dogs, is a highly aggressive hematological tumor with 2 to 8 weeks of expected life from diagnosis [Lawman *et al.*, 2008].

The use of hGM-CSF secreting autologous tumor cell vaccine was safe, but it did not result in clinical benefit for canine B-cell lymphoma patients [Turek *et al.*, 2007].

In another *ex vivo* approach, Emm55 a Streptococcus pyogenes serotyping antigen gene was transferred to autologous tumor cells of 7 canine lymphoma patients [Lawman *et al.*, 2008]. Once treated, all of them developed an antibody response to multiple autologous tumor antigens and CD8+ mediated cellular cytotoxicity. One long lasting complete response (>18 months) and 3 extended survivals support further trials. No adverse effects related to treatment were informed.

Peruzzi *et al.* [2010] proposed a vaccine against dog telomerase reverse transcriptase (dTERT) as a valid target for immunotherapy of malignant lymphoma when combined with standard chemotherapy regimen. dTERT-specific immune response was induced in 13 out of 14 treated animals (93%) and remained detectable and long-lasting with the absence of autoimmunity or other side effects. Most interestingly, the survival time of vaccine/chemo-treated dogs was significantly increased over historic controls of chemo-treated animals (>97.8 versus 37 weeks).

A completely different strategy that also can be considered as RNA mediated gene therapy was proposed by Sorenmo *et al.* [2011] to treat non-Hodgkin's lymphoma. In that case, when administered to dogs in remission after induction chemotherapy, *ex vivo* autologous tumor RNA electroporated CD40-activated B cells, safely stimulated immunity *in vivo*. This approach was safe and potentiated the effects of salvage therapy, improving the rate of durable second remissions as well as subsequent lymphoma-specific survival following salvage therapy.

Other Canine Tumors and Therapy Approaches

As reported by Reed *et al.* [2010] electrochemogene therapy (ECGT) combining electroporation with a feline IL-12 carrying plasmid and bleomycin was very effective. It controlled two oral squamous cell carcinoma and one acanthomatous ameloblastoma tumor that displayed long lasting complete responses (56, 27 and 9 months tumor-free, respectively).

An astrocytoma bearing patient was treated by a combination of surgery, intracavitary adenoviral interferon-γ gene transfer, and vaccination with glioma cell lysates mixed with CpG oligodeoxynucleotides [Pluhar *et al.*, 2010]. Transient neurological symptoms resolved and this dog remained tumor-free over 450 days following surgery.

Even though they did not aimed to fight directly against cancer, Draghia-Akli *et al.* [2002] successfully contributed in diminishing paraneoplastic symptoms in canine patients with advanced melanoma, sarcoma, carcinoma and lymphoma. By *in vivo* electroporation enhanced delivery of a plasmid containing the growth hormone releasing hormone (GHRH) gene, they succeeded in normalizing the hematological parameters. In a larger controlled trial, they showed that responder dogs survived 84% longer than nonresponders and controls [Bodles-Brakhop *et al.*, 2008]. The quality of life, defined by 10 different parameters, dramatically improved with treatment.

Two feasibility studies for viral gene transfer to tumors using marker genes were reported. Chauvet *et al.* [1998] demonstrated that intra-arterial (carotid) injection of adenoviral vector could be used to transfer genes to a benign canine meningioma. Dumey *et al.* [2005], using intravesical instillation of retroviral vector were able to selectively transfer genes into canine malignant bladder tumors.

Conclusion

Most of the veterinary cancer gene therapy trials on patients with spontaneous tumors could be classified as immunogene therapy and were performed with non-viral vectors. In general terms very slight or no adverse collateral effects were found and most of the times treated animals displayed a better course of the disease (longer survival, delayed or suppressed local or systemic relapse, recovery of the quality of life) suggesting the utility of this sort of strategy as standard adjuvant treatment.

Two emerging approaches are supported by a large number of treated patients: the xenogeneic vaccine developed by Bergman *et al.* [2003], and the suicide gene plus autologous/allogeneic vaccine developed by Finocchiaro and Glikin [2008a]. Both systems based the systemic disease control on the immune system. While the first approach using hTyr vaccine was specific for melanoma [Grosenbaugh *et al.* 2011], the second approach appeared to be more versatile, because it was successfully translated to other kinds of tumors such as soft tissue sarcoma [Finocchiaro *et al.* 2011] and osteosarcoma [Finocchiaro *et al.* 2012].

Besides, all these trials also demonstrate the utility of spontaneous tumors in companion animals as a valid translational model for the evaluation of novel DNA based therapies.

As it is the case for human patients, usually survival times for those veterinary patients that displayed objectives responses were significantly higher than for non responders. In addition better results were obtained when treating the early stages of the disease and, in the case of advanced disease presenting bulky tumors, previous standard procedures such as surgery, chemotherapy and/or radiotherapy were necessary to obtain the best outcome of the whole treatment.

It is worth to note that the efficacy displayed by plasmid-based non-viral vectors used in 80% of the trials involving large animals demonstrated their usefulness for present and future gene therapy treatments.

Although intravenous injections of cationic lipid:DNA complexes had some anti-tumor activity against canine STS regardless the transgene carried by the plasmid in the case of angiostatin "therapeutic" or luciferase "reporter" gene [Kamstock *et al.*, 2006], this fact should no be taken as negative. In addition to the immune enhancing effects of complexes carrying non-coding plasmid in a vaccine proposed against hemangiosarcoma [U'Ren *et al.*, 2007], the expression of therapeutic genes displayed specific anti-tumor activity as repeatedly evidenced in many papers listed in Table 1. Further work has to be done to ascertain the contribution of each component *in vivo*.

An increasing interest in cancer therapy trials in large animals (especially dogs and cats) including those using gene therapy techniques will serve as concept, safety and effectiveness proofs. This new trend in the research of novel cancer therapies will indeed benefit both companion animals and human patients [Hansen *et al.* 2006, Paoloni and Khanna 2007].

Table 1. Canine cancer gene therapy trials

#	TUMOR / *Approach*	GENE	VECTOR	MODE	RESULTS	AUTHORS / YEAR
1	MEL *Im-Ther*	hIL-2	Irradiated hIL-2 producing xenogeneic cells made by plasmid transfection	*Ex vivo – p.t.*	(n=16) NR, 480 d. Control: 1 / Treated: 6 Median Survival: Treated: 270 d / Control: 75 d	Quintin-Colonna *et al.* 1996
2	MEL FSA OSA HGS *Im-Ther*	hGM-CSF	Irradiated hGM-CSF producing autologous tumor cells plasmid transferred by gene gun	*Ex vivo – i.d.*	MEL (n=10) 1 CR (300 d), 1 PR (300 d), 1 NED (250 d), 1 SD (125 d) FSA (n=3) 1 PR, 1 NED (175 d)	Hogge *et al.* 1998
3	MGA *Marker*	EcLac Z	Adenovirus	*In vivo – i.a.*	(n=1) Feasibility study: successful marker expression	Chauvet *et al.* 1998
4	MEL *Im-Ther*	Enterotoxin-B + cGM-CSF	Plasmid lipofection:	*In vivo – i.t. / p.t. / i.l.n.*	(n=12) Median survival (stage III): Treated: 168 d / Hist. surgery controls: 105 d	Dow *et al.* 1998
5	CAR STS LYP *Other*	mpGHRH	Naked plasmid electroporation	*In vivo – i.m.*	At 56 d, treated (n=16) improved hematological parameters compared to control (n=19)	Draghia-Akli *et al.* 2002
6	STS *Im-Ther*	Enterotoxin-A + cIL-2	Plasmid lipofection:	*In vivo – i.t.*	(n=16) 3 CR, 1 PR, 1 SD (84 d). Responders survival > 540 d w/o relapse.	Thamm *et al.* 2003
7	MEL *Im-Ther*	hTyr	Naked plasmid – Jet injection	*In vivo – i.m.*	(n=9) 1 CR, 2 NED, 1 SD (14 d) / Median survival: 389 d. Hist. controls (s II 150 d, s III 60 d). Humoral antibod.: 3/9. (n=58) Median survival: >750 d. Hist. controls: 324 d.	Bergman *et al.* 2003 Liao *et al.* 2006 Grosenbaugh *et al.* 2011
8	MEL *Pro-Apop*	hFasL	Plasmid lipofection:	*In vivo – i.t.*	(n=5) GT: 3 TR, 1 SD / CT: 2 CR, 2 PR Survival: 168-574 d	Bianco *et al.* 2003
9	MEL *Im-Ther*	hgp100	Autologous Adenovirus transduced dendritic cells	*Ex vivo – s.c.*	(n=3) survival ranging 210 - 1440 d	Gyorffy *et al.* 2005

#	TUMOR / *Approach*	GENE	VECTOR	MODE	RESULTS	AUTHORS / YEAR
10	OSA – lung metastases *Im-Ther*	cIL-2	Plasmid lipofection:	*In vivo – i.v.*	(n=20) 84 d: 1 CR, 2 PR, 4 SD. Median survival (s IV): Treated: 82 d / Hist. surgery controls: 58 d	Dow *et al.* 2005
11	MBT *Marker*	nlsLacZ neo^R	Retrovirus	*In vivo – i.v.i.*	Feasibility study: successful marker expression.	Dumey *et al.* 2005
12	MEL *Im-Ther*	hTyr / mTyr mgp75 hGM-CSF	Naked plasmid – Jet injection	*In vivo – i.m.*	Different combinations and doses. Median survival Stages II-III (n=33) w/ locoregional control: 569 d. 25/33 still alive.	Bergman *et al.* 2006
13	MEL *Im-Ther*	hgp100	Irradiated allogeneic hgp100 expressing tumor cells plasmid transferred by gene gun	*Ex vivo – i.d.*	(n=34) Median survival: Responders (CR,PR,SD) (n=12), 337 d / Non-responders (n=20), 95 d	Alexander *et al.* 2006
14	LYP *Im-Ther*	hGM-CSF	Plasmid lipofection:	*In vivo – i.d.*	Vaccine (n=26) / Placebo (n=26). Median survival 474 d	Turek *et al.* 2007
15	MEL *Suic-G + Im-Ther*	HSV-*tk* hIL-2 hGM-CSF	Plasmid lipofection: HSV-*tk* + GCV. Irradiated xenogeneic hIL-2 and hGM-CSF producing cells made by plasmid lipofection	*In vivo (SG) – i.t. / Ex vivo (CPXC) – i.t.*	Combined treatment (n=45) / Surgery controls (n=23). Median survival: 160 d / 82 d. Metastasis-free median survival: >509 d / 133 d. Combined treatment: CR=16%, PR=31%, SD=27%, PD=27%.	Finocchiaro *et al.* 2008.
16	MEL *Suic-G + Im-Ther*	HSV-*tk* hIL-2 hGM-CSF	Plasmid lipofection: HSV-*tk* + GCV. Irradiated xenogeneic hIL-2 and hGM-CSF producing cells made by plasmid lipofection	*In vivo (SG) - i.t. / Ex vivo (CPXC)+ (TV) – s.c.*	Combined treatment (n=100) / Surgery controls (n=51): Local disease-free patients: 58% / 6%. Metastasis-free patients: 78% / 43%. Median survival: >1312 d / 78 d. Metastasis-free median survival: >1312 d / 112 d.	Finocchiaro and Glikin. 2008
17	MEL *Im-Ther*	CD40L	Adenovirus	*In vivo – i.t.*	(n=2) Feasible and manageable toxicity 1 NED 401 d 1 PR >150 d	von Euler *et al.* 2008

Table 1. (Continued)

#	TUMOR / *Approach*	GENE	VECTOR	MODE	RESULTS	AUTHORS / YEAR
18	HGS CAR STS ADC MCT MEL *Other*	mpGHRH	Naked plasmid electroporation	*In vivo – i.m.*	54.2 % responses at day 90 (n=43). Responders lived 84 % more than non responders.	Bodles-Brakhop *et al.* 2008
19	LYP ***Im-Ther***	Emm55	Plasmid/electroporation	*Ex vivo – i.v.*	(n=7) 1 CR > 555 d, 6 PR, 3 extended survival > 2X	Lawman *et al.* 2008
20	ASC ***Im-Ther***	IFN-γ	Adenovirus	*In vivo – p.t* *+ (TV) – s.c*	(n=1) Feasible. Disease-free survival > 450 d	Pluhar *et al.* 2010
21	SCC AMB MEL STS ***Im-Ther***	fIL-12	Naked plasmid + bleomycin + electroporation	*In vivo – i.t*	n=5 2 SSC and AMB resolved (56, 27, 9 months tumor-free).	Reed *et al.* 2010
22	LYP ***Im-Ther***	cTERT-LTB cTERT	Naked plasmid electroporation + Adenovirus 6	*In vivo – i.m.*	(n=14) GT + Chemo (n=8) Chemo. Median survival: >96 wks / 28 wks. Time to first relapse: >26 wks/ 12 wks.	Peruzzi *et al.* 2010
23	MEL Digital ***Im-Ther***	mTyr	Naked plasmid – Jet injection	*In vivo – i.m.*	(n=58) Median survival: >476 d Surgery only historical controls: 365d	Manley *et al.* 2011

#	TUMOR / Approach	GENE	VECTOR	*MODE*	RESULTS	AUTHORS / YEAR
24	LYP ***Im-Ther***	cNHL-mRNA	NHL-mRNA loaded electroporation	*Ex vivo RNA* transfer *In vivo* Chemo.	(n=19) significant lymphoma-specific survival following salvage therapy	Sorenmo *et al.* 2011
25	STS OSA ***Suic-G*** + ***Im-Ther***	HSV-*tk* IFN-β hIL-2 hGM-CSF	Plasmid lipofection: HSV-*tk* + IFN-β + GCV. Irradiated xenogeneic hIL-2 and hGM-CSF producing cells made by plasmid lipofection	*In vivo (SG) + (IFN-β) - i.t. / Ex vivo (CPXC) + (TV) – s.c*	STS (n=11) 5 survived > 2 years, 4 survived > 1 year OSA (n=6) 2 survived > 1 year	Finocchiaro *et al.* 2011 Finocchiaro *et al.* 2012

ADC, Adenocarcinoma; AMB, acanthomatous ameloblastoma; ASC, astrocytoma; CAR, carcinoma; FSA, fibrosarcoma; HGS, hemangiosarcoma; LYP, lymphoma; MBT, malignant bladder tumors; MEL, melanoma; MCT, mast cell tumor; MEL: melanoma; MGA, meningioma; OSA, osteosarcoma; SCC, squamous cell carcinoma; STS, soft tissue sarcoma // ***Im-Ther***, immunotherapy; ***Pro-Apop***, proapoptotic; ***Suic-G***, suicide gene // CD40L, CD40 ligand; cGM-CSF, canine granulocyte macrophage colony stimulating factor; cIL-2, canine interleukin-2; cNHL-mRNA: non-Hodgin lymphoma RNA; TERT, canine telomerase reverse transcriptase; EcLacZ, *E. col*i lacZ; Emm55, *streptococcus pyogenes* serotyping; antigen; fIL-12, feline interleukin-12; hFasL, human Fas ligand; hGM-CSF, human granulocyte macrophage colony stimulating factor; hgp100, human glycoprotein 100; hIL-2, human interleukin-2; HSV-*tk*, herpes simplex thymidine kinase; hTyr, human tyrosinase; IFN-γ, interferon-γ; LTB, *E. coli* heat labile enterotoxin; mgp75, mouse glycoprotein 75; mpGHRH, mutated porcine growth hormone releasing hormone; mTyr, mouse tyrosinase; neo^R, neomycin resistance gene; nlsLacZ, *E. coli* lacZ with nuclear localization sequence // CR, complete response; NED, no evidence of disease; NR, no relapse; PR, partial response; SD, steady disease // Chemo, chemotherapy; CPXC, cytokine producing xenogeneic cells; GCV, ganciclovir; SG, suicide gene; TV, tumor vaccine; *i.a.*, intra-arterial; *i.d.*, intradermal; *i.l.n.*, intra-lymph node; *i.m.*, intramuscular, *i.t.*, intratumoral; *i.v.*, intravenous; *i.v.i.*, intra-vesical instillation; *p.t.*, peritumoral; *s.c.*, subcutaneous // d, days; Hist, historical; wks, weeks.

Trials in companion animals are shorter in time and at lower costs than in humans. Nowadays, there are conditions for the development of translational research in the oncology field [Porrello *et al.*, 2004], intending to apply scientific information to solve present problems in relatively brief periods of time. Proper cancer models involving companion animals spontaneously induce the investigators to work in the duality between the veterinary perspective and the potential application to human medicine. However, these are not contradictory objectives, and trials in humans based on the equivalent trials in pets will possibly come soon.

Acknowledgments

This work was partially supported by grants: ANPCYT-FONCYT PICT2007-00539, CONICET PIP2009-112 200801 02920 and UBACYT PID2011-200 201001 00504. G.C.G. and L.M.E.F. are investigators of the Consejo Nacional de Investigaciones Científicas y Técnicas (CONICET, Argentina).

References

Alexander AN, Huelsmeyer MK, Mitzey A, Dubielzig RR, Kurzman ID, MacEwen EG, Vail DM. Development of an allogeneic whole-cell tumor vaccine expressing xenogeneic gp100 and its implementation in a phase II clinical trial in canine patients with malignant melanoma. *Cancer Immunol Immunother.* 2006, *55:* 433-442.

Bergman PJ, Camps-Palau MA, McKnight JA, Leibman NF, Craft DM, Leung C, Liao J, Riviere I, Sadelain M, Hohenhaus AE, *et al.* Development of a xenogeneic DNA vaccine program for canine malignant melanoma at the Animal Medical Center. *Vaccine.* 2006; *24:* 4582-4585.

Bergman PJ, McKnight J, Novosad A, Charney S, Farrelly J, Craft D, Wulderk M, Jeffers Y, Sadelain M, Hohenhaus AE, *et al.* Long-term survival of dogs with advanced malignant melanoma after DNA vaccination with xenogeneic human tyrosinase: a phase I trial. *Clin. Cancer Res.* 2003; *9:* 1284-1290.

Bianco SR, Sun J, Fosmire SP, Hance K, Padilla ML, Ritt MG, Getzy DM, Duke RC, Withrow SJ, Lana S, Matthiesen DT, *et al.* Enhancing antimelanoma immune responses through apoptosis. *Cancer Gene Ther.* 2003; *10:* 726-736.

Bodles-Brakhop AM, Brown PA, Pope MA, Draghia-Akli R. Double-blinded, Placebo-controlled plasmid GHRH trial for cancer-associated anemia in dogs. *Mol. Ther.* 2008; *16:* 862-70.

Casal M, Haskins M. Large animal models and gene therapy. *Eur. J. Hum. Genet.* 2006; *14:* 266-272.

Chauvet AE, Kesava PP, Goh CS, Badie B. Selective intraarterial gene delivery into a canine meningioma. *J. Neurosurg.* 1998; *88:* 870-873.

Dow S, Elmslie R, Kurzman I, MacEwen G, Pericle F, Liggitt D. Phase I study of liposome-DNA complexes encoding the interleukin-2 gene in dogs with osteosarcoma lung metastases. *Hum. Gene Ther.* 2005; *16:* 937-946.

Dow SW, Elmslie RE, Willson AP, Roche L, Gorman C, Potter TA. In vivo tumor transfection with superantigen plus cytokine genes induces tumor regression and prolongs survival in dogs with malignant melanoma. *J. Clin. Invest.* 1998; *101:* 2406-2414.

Draghia-Akli R, Hahn KA, King GK, Cummings KK, Carpenter RH. Effects of plasmid-mediated growth hormone-releasing hormone in severely debilitated dogs with cancer. *Mol. Ther.* 2002; *6:* 830-836.

Dumey N, Mongiat-Artus P, Devauchelle P, Lesourd A, Cotard JP, Le Duc A, Marty M, Cussenot O, Cohen-Haguenauer O. In vivo retroviral mediated gene transfer into bladder urothelium results in preferential transduction of tumoral cells. *Eur. Urol.* 2005; *47:* 257-263.

Ehrhart N. Soft-tissue sarcomas in dogs: a review. *J. Am. Anim. Hosp. Assoc.* 2005; *41:* 241-246.

Finocchiaro LME, Fiszman GL, Karara AL, Glikin GC. Suicide gene and cytokines combined non viral gene therapy for canine spontaneous melanoma. *Cancer Gene Ther.* 2008; *15:* 165-172.

Finocchiaro LME, Glikin GC. Cancer gene therapy in large animals. In *New Gene Therapy and Cancer Research,* W.B. Gustafsson (Ed.). Nova Science Publishers, Inc. (New York, U.S.A.). pp. 279-292 (2008). ISBN: 1-60021-969-1.[b]

Finocchiaro LME, Glikin GC. Cytokine-enhanced vaccine and suicide gene therapy as surgery adjuvant treatments for spontaneous canine melanoma. *Gene Ther.* 2008; *15:* 267-276.[a]

Finocchiaro LME, Spector A, Rossi UA, Gil-Cardeza ML, Suarez JL, Riveros MD, Villaverde MS, Glikin GC. The potential of suicide plus immune gene therapy for treating osteosarcoma: the experience on canine veterinary patients. In *Sarcoma: Symptoms, Causes and Treatments.* E.J.

Butler (Ed.). Nova Science Publishers, Inc. (New York, U.S.A.), (2012). ISBN: 978-1-62100-362-5. In press.

Finocchiaro, LME, Villaverde, MS, Gil-Cardeza, ML, Riveros, MD, Glikin, GC. Cytokine-enhanced vaccine and interferon-β plus suicide gene as combined therapy for spontaneous canine sarcomas. *Res. Vet. Sci.* 2011, *91*, 230-234.

Grosenbaugh DA, Leard AT, Bergman PJ, Klein MK, Meleo K, Susaneck S, Hess PR, Jankowski MK, Jones PD, Leibman NF et al. Safety and efficacy of a xenogeneic DNA vaccine encoding for human tyrosinase as adjunctive treatment for oral malignant melanoma in dogs following surgical excision of the primary tumor. *Am. J. Vet. Res.* 2011; *72:* 1631-8.

Gyorffy S, Rodriguez-Lecompte JC, Woods JP, Foley R, Kruth S, Liaw PC, Gauldie J. Bone marrow-derived dendritic cell vaccination of dogs with naturally occurring melanoma by using human gp100 antigen. *J. Vet. Intern. Med.* 2005; *19:* 56-63.

Hansen K, Khanna C. Spontaneous and genetically engineered animal models; use in preclinical cancer drug development. *Eur. J. Cancer.* 2004; *40:* 858-880.

Hogge GS, Burkholder JK, Culp J, Albertini MR, Dubielzig RR, Keller ET, Yang NS, MacEwen EG. Development of human granulocyte-macrophage colony-stimulating factor-transfected tumor cell vaccines for the treatment of spontaneous canine cancer. *Hum. Gene Ther.* 1998; *9:* 1851-1861.

Kamstock D, Guth A, Elmslie R, Kurzman I, Liggitt D, Coro L, Fairman J, Dow S Liposome-DNA complexes infused intravenously inhibit tumor angiogenesis and elicit antitumor activity in dogs with soft tissue sarcoma. *Cancer Gene Ther.* 2006; *13:* 306-317.

Lawman M, Eidizadeh S, Selmon C, Kane C, Xigacos L, Kaufman L, Shaw N, Lawman P. Anti-tumor response induced by autologous cancer vaccine in canine lymphoma. *Cancer Ther.* 2008, *6:* 827-840,

Liao JC, Gregor P, Wolchok JD, Orlandi F, Craft D, Leung C, Houghton AN, Bergman PJ. Vaccination with human tyrosinase DNA induces antibody responses in dogs with advanced melanoma. *Cancer Immun.* 2006; *6:* 8.

MacEwen EG, Kurzman ID, Vail DM, Dubielzig RR, Everlith K, Madewell BR, Rodriguez CO Jr, Phillips B, Zwahlen CH, Obradovich J *et al.* Adjuvant therapy for melanoma in dogs: results of randomized clinical trials using surgery, liposome-encapsulated muramyl tripeptide, and granulocyte macrophage colony-stimulating factor. *Clin. Cancer Res.* 1999; *5:* 4249-4258)

Manley CA, Leibman NF, Wolchok JD, Rivière IC, Bartido S, Craft DM, Bergman PJ. Xenogeneic murine tyrosinase DNA vaccine for malignant melanoma of the digit of dogs. *J. Vet. Intern. Med.* 2011; *25:* 94-99.

Mayer MN, Grier CK. Palliative radiation therapy for canine osteosarcoma. *Can. Vet. J.* 2006; *47:* 707-709.

Ohlfest JR, Freese AB, Largaespada DA. Nonviral vectors for cancer gene therapy: prospects for integrating vectors and combination therapies. *Curr. Gene Ther.* 2005; *5:* 629-641.

Paoloni MC, Khanna C. Comparative oncology today. *Vet. Clin. North Am. Small Anim. Pract.* 2007; *37:* 1023-1032.

Peruzzi D, Gavazza A, Mesiti G, Lubas G, Scarselli E, Conforti A, Bendtsen C, Ciliberto G, La Monica N, Aurisicchio L. A vaccine targeting telomerase enhances survival of dogs affected by B-cell lymphoma. *Mol. Ther.* 2010; *18:* 1559-67.

Pluhar GE, Grogan PG, Seiler C, Goulart M, Santacruz KS, Carlson C, Chen W, Olin MR, Lowenstein PR, Castro MG, Haines SJ, Ohlfest JR. Anti-tumor immune response correlates with neurological symptoms in a dog with spontaneous astrocytoma treated by gene and vaccine therapy. *Vaccine* 2010; *28:* 3371-3378.

Porrello A, Cardelli P, Spugnini EP. Pet models in cancer research: general principles. *J. Exp. Clin. Cancer Res.* 2004; *23:* 181-193.

Quintin-Colonna F, Devauchelle P, Fradelizi D, Mourot B, Faure T, Kourilsky P, Roth C, Mehtali M. Gene therapy of spontaneous canine melanoma and feline fibrosarcoma by intratumoral administration of histoincompatible cells expressing human interleukin-2. *Gene Ther.* 1996; *3:* 1104-1112.

Reed SD, Fulmer A, Buckholz J, Zhang B, Cutrera J, Shiomitsu K, Li S. Bleomycin/ interleukin-12 electrochemogene therapy for treating naturally occurring spontaneous neoplasms in dogs. *Cancer Gene Ther.* 2010; 17: 457-64.

Rosenberg SA, Aebersold P, Cornetta K, Kasid A, Morgan RA, Moen R, Karson EM, Lotze MT, Yang JC, Topalian SL, *et al.* Gene transfer into humans--immunotherapy of patients with advanced melanoma, using tumor-infiltrating lymphocytes modified by retroviral gene transduction. *N. Engl. J. Med.* 1990; *323:* 570-578.

Sorenmo KU, Krick E, Coughlin CM, Overley B, Gregor TP, Vonderheide RH, Mason NJ. CD40-activated B cell cancer vaccine improves second clinical remission and survival in privately owned dogs with non-Hodgkin's lymphoma. *PLoS One.* 2011; *6:* e24167.

Thamm DH, Kurzman ID, MacEwen EG, Feinmehl R, Towell TL, Longhofer SL, Johnson CM, Geoly FJ, Stinchcomb DT. Intralesional lipid-complexed cytokine/superantigen immunogene therapy for spontaneous canine tumors. *Cancer Immunol Immunother.* 2003; *52:* 473-480.

Turek MM, Thamm DH, Mitzey A, Kurzman ID, Huelsmeyer MK, Dubielzig RR, Vail DM. Human granulocyte-macrophage colony-stimulating factor DNA cationic-lipid complexed autologous tumour cell vaccination in the treatment of canine B-cell multicentric lymphoma. *Vet. Comp. Oncol.* 2007; *5*: 219–231.

U'Ren LW, Biller BJ, Elmslie RE, Thamm DH, Dow SW. Evaluation of a novel tumor vaccine in dogs with hemangiosarcoma. *J. Vet. Intern. Med.* 2007; 21:113-120.

Vail DM, MacEwen EG. Spontaneously occurring tumors of companion animals as models for human cancer. *Cancer Invest.* 2000; *18*: 781-792.

Vassaux G, Groot-Wassink T. In vivo noninvasive imaging for gene therapy. J. *Biomed. Biotechnol.* 2003: 92-101.

von Euler H, Sadeghi A, Carlsson B, Rivera P, Loskog A, Segall T, Korsgren O, Tötterman TH. Efficient adenovector CD40 ligand immunotherapy of canine malignant melanoma. *J. Immunother.* 2008, *31*: 377-384.

In: Canine Behavior, Classification and Diseases ISBN: 978-1-62081-304-1
Editors: R. L. Andrade and C. I. Batista

Chapter III

Canine Carcinogenesis in Translational Cancer Research

Salomé S. Pinho[1,2], Sandra Carvalho[1,2], Joana Cabral[1], Celso A. Reis[1,2,3] and Fátima Gärtner[1,2]

[1]Institute of Molecular Pathology and Immunology of the University of Porto (IPATIMUP), Portugal

[2]Institute of Biomedical Sciences of Abel Salazar (ICBAS), University of Porto, Portugal

[3]Medical Faculty, University of Porto, Portugal

Abstract

The biological complexity of human cancer has stimulated the development of complex experimental systems that could resemble in a natural and spontaneous manner the physiopathological aspects of cancer biology. Companion animals display many aspects of the complexity of human cancer filling the gap between *in vitro* and *in vivo* studies. Spontaneous tumors in dogs share a wide variety of epidemiological, biological and clinical features with human cancer, which makes this a valid tumor model system available for studying cancer biology in oncology research. In this review we summarize the importance of naturally occurring canine tumors as a valuable model for studying many aspects of human cancer, as well as the potential use of this animal model for the development of new cancer treatments.

Introduction

Cancer is a highly complex biological process that requires appropriate experimental model systems for studying the intricate aspects and steps of its development and progression (Hanahan and Weinberg 2011). The ideal experimental model for cancer research should reproduce as close as possible the biochemical, molecular and genetic pathways, histological and physiological features, and the metastatic patterns of cancer biology (Alison 2004; Cespedes, Casanova et al. 2006). Different in vitro and in vivo models are available in oncology research. Spontaneous tumors in dogs are considered a valuable and appropriate tool for studying numerous aspects of human cancer with mutual benefits. In this chapter we will summarize the importance of canine tumors in translational cancer research giving a systems biology approach by focusing on genomics; proteomics and glycomics comparative aspects of both human and canine.

Models for Cancer Research: *In Vitro* Models

The use of in vitro tumorigenic cell line models has enabled the study of important molecular aspects of carcinogenesis. In vitro models allow controlled conditions and reproducible results enabling the validation, repetition, and optimization of the experimental assays. Furthermore, in vitro assays are relatively inexpensive, associated to high throughput, and are unconstrained by the practical ethical considerations required with in vivo models (Masters 2002; Gordon and Khanna 2010).

However, in vitro cancer models do not closely mimic important features of human cancer. The growth of tumor cell lines occurs in a bi-dimensional context and is promoted by an artificial environment. These conditions lead to the selection of phenotypic characteristics favorable to the in vitro growth, namely selection of clones with a given set of gene expressions, morphological and functional properties. In addition, in vitro studies do not take in account the tumor microenvironment and host-tumor interactions, which are crucial in cancer progression and response to therapy (Masters 2002; Gordon and Khanna 2010; Hanahan and Weinberg 2011; Pinho 2012) .

Models for Cancer Research: Murine Models

Murine models have been a fundamental tool in the study of the complexity of human cancer providing valuable insights in cancer biology. These models gather many advantages in cancer research such as their relatively small sizes, propensity to breed in captivity, short gestation times and also their similarities in organ systems, systemic physiology and genes with human counterpart. Furthermore, and unlike *in vitro* models, murine models allow the three-dimensional growth of tumors with direct interaction with the stromal microenvironment (Gordon and Khanna 2010; Rowell, McCarthy et al. 2011). The *in vivo* experiments are essential to understand the fundamental mechanisms underpinning malignancy and to discover improved methods to prevent, diagnose and treat cancer. All experiments should be conducted incorporating the 3Rs: replacement, reduction and refinement, according to the EU guidelines for the welfare and use of animals in cancer research.

The murine models that are most often used in cancer research are the xenografts and the genetically engineered mouse (GEM). The orthotopic xenograft of human tumors provides realistic heterogeneity of tumor cells and can predict the drug response of a tumor in a human patient. However, these mice models are immunocompromised, so their immune system and their stromal and vascular components are not syngeneic (Voskoglou-Nomikos, Pater et al. 2003; Hansen and Khanna 2004; Becher and Holland 2006; Richmond and Su 2008). In GEM models, the genetic profile can be altered by mutation, deletion or overexpression of one or several genes though to be involved in cancer process. Therefore, GEM models provide the opportunity to test the role of a specific set of human genes and proteins within an *in vivo* context, and to follow tumor development from early time points in a realistic microenvironment. GEMs are histologically and genetically more accurate models of human cancer than xenografts (Hansen and Khanna 2004; Becher and Holland 2006; Richmond and Su 2008). Nevertheless, the murine models have some disadvantages in cancer research. In mouse models, the carcinogenic process is often artificially induced and not arises spontaneously as it occurs in human. In addition, the genetic manipulation of mouse models, as mentioned above, involves one or few genes, being therefore missed the gene networks and interactions that are crucial for cancer development and progression (Rowell, McCarthy et al. 2011). Other relevant biological differences between transplanted tumors in mice models and naturally occurring cancers in humans include telomerase that is functionally active in most murine cells; the alterations of certain genes sets and pathways that can vary between murine and human cells; the fact that mice can tolerate higher concentrations of drugs and proteins than human patients, and that murine bone marrow may be less sensitive to many cytotoxic agents. In summary, the process of tumor development and progression observed in mouse models are not predictive of what happens in human with tumors of same histology which restricts the translation of the scientific advances from preclinical studies to improved treatments for patients with cancer (Rangarajan and Weinberg 2003; Hansen and Khanna 2004; Teicher 2009). Therefore, there is a growing need for more predictive and informative pre-clinical cancer models that more faithfully mimic many aspects of the complexity of human cancer.

Canine as Models for Cancer Research

Companion animals (pet dogs and cats) seem to have many of the desired characteristics that fill the gap between *in vitro* and *in vivo* models (Pinho 2012). Naturally occurring tumors in dogs have many epidemiological, biological, clinical, histological, genetic and molecular similarities to human cancers that are difficult to replicate using other model systems (MacEwen 1990).

The types of cancer observed in pet dogs with potential relevance for human cancer biology studies include melanoma, non-Hodgkin lymphoma (NHL), leukaemia, osteosarcoma, soft tissue sarcomas, prostate, mammary, nasal, lung, bladder and gastrointestinal carcinomas, among others.

One of the most important features of canines as valuable comparative models for human cancer research is the spontaneous nature of the carcinogenic process that develops in the environment of an intact immune system where the surrounding stroma is syngeneic. In addition, most of these tumors are often driven by genetic and/or molecular dysfunctions similarly to human tumors. The recent release of the entire canine genome sequence showed that for many genes families and particular those associated with cancer high homology and close similarity with the human gene sequences have been found to be much closer than the respective counterparts in mouse (Paoloni and Khanna 2008; Gordon and Khanna 2010).

There is a growing interest of cancer researchers in canine models that has been accompanied by the increasing number of publications in veterinary oncology research, which makes comparative oncology of utmost importance in translational medicine and ultimately in clinical application (De Vico, Maiolino et al. 2005; Paoloni and Khanna 2008; Pinho 2012).

Canine Tumors as a Mirror of Human Cancer: Mammary Carcinogenesis as Example

Mammary gland tumors are the most common neoplasia of female dogs. Similarly, breast cancer is the second leading cause of cancer-related death in women after lung cancer and is the most common cancer among women.

Canine mammary tumors have many similarities with woman breast cancer that arise from the comparable tumor genesis, progression and metastatic process. In addition, there is a close homology between canine and human signaling pathways, gene sets and molecular mechanisms that are known to be important in mammary carcinogenesis (Klopfleisch, von Euler et al. 2011; Pinho 2012). Contrasting to laboratory rodents, dogs share a mutual environment with people and, consequently, may be exposed to some of the same carcinogens (Knapp and Waters 1997; Vail and MacEwen 2000). Dogs are more outbred than laboratory rodents, yet certain breeds are at increased risk for developing mammary tumors (Knapp and Waters 1997). Furthermore, dogs have a shorter life span than people; it is possible to study mammary carcinomas that develop after a few years instead of decades. Therefore, canine mammary tumors have been considered a powerful comparative and predictive model of woman breast cancer.

Genomics, Proteomics and Signaling Pathways: A Comparative Analysis

It has been demonstrated the existence of a significant overlap between canine and human genes and signaling pathways that play a role in the process of tumor development and progression (Pinho, Reis et al. 2009; Pinho 2012). It was recently demonstrated that many genes deregulated in human breast cancer were also found to be deregulated in canine mammary tumors compared with normal mammary tissue. This first genome-wide comparative analysis showed that the pathways showing to be upregulated in tumors from both species are those related to increased proliferation activity, whereas the pathways related to cell development, cell-matrix adhesion and cell-cell communication are downregulated. Furthermore, it was also demonstrated a high homology between human and canine mammary tumors in the perturbation of many cancer-related signaling pathways such as PI3K/AKR, KRAS, Wnt- β-catenin, and MAPK cascade and in cancer-related gene sets (Uva, Aurisicchio et al. 2009).

The PI3K/AKT signaling pathway plays a critical role in the regulation of cellular growth, proliferation, and survival. The activation of oncogenes and/or inactivation of suppressor genes disrupt the signaling equilibrium and can thus lead to cellular transformation, namely to the development of breast cancer. In human breast cancer, the expression of activating point mutations at phosphoinositide-3-kinase catalytic alpha polypeptide (PIK3CA), the loss of PTEN activity, and mutation of v-akt-murine thymoma viral oncogene homolog 1 (AKT1) are associated with aberrant PI3K pathway signaling. The dysregulation of the PI3K/Akt pathway in human cancer is associated with poor prognosis, highlighting the enormous potential impact on patient survival that the inhibition of this pathway could achieve (Dillon, White et al. 2007; Saal, Johansson et al. 2007; Galanis, Pappa et al. 2008; Castaneda, Cortes-Funes et al. 2010). In canine mammary tumors, the PI3K/ AKT signaling pathway has a similar molecular dysregulation as in human breast cancer (Uva, Aurisicchio et al. 2009; Pinho 2012).

KRAS is an oncogene involved in a cancer-related pathway that is similarly upregulated in human breast cancer and canine mammary tumors (Sweet-Cordero, Mukherjee et al. 2005; Uva, Aurisicchio et al. 2009).

MAPK cascade is associated with the response to extracellular stimuli, regulation of gene expression, mitosis, differentiation, cell survival and apoptosis, and is also equally upregulated in both human and canine mammary tumors (Sebolt-Leopold and Herrera 2004; Uva, Aurisicchio et al. 2009).

The gatekeeper tumor suppressor gene PTEN is involved in numerous mechanisms that lead to cellular defense against neoplastic transformation and progression. It was demonstrated loss of PTEN expression in human breast cancer (Saal, Johansson et al. 2007; Milovanovic, Dzodic et al. 2011; Singh, Odriozola et al. 2011). Similarly, in canine mammary tumor it was demonstrated that PTEN expression is decreased in mammary tumor cells.

Therefore, PTEN can be considered a useful prognostic marker in mammary tumors (Ressel, Millanta et al. 2009).

BRCA1 and BRCA2 genes are critical players in the maintenance of genome stability, being involved in DNA damage response, repair and recombination, checkpoint control of cell cycle, and transcription (Venkitaraman 2002). The dysregulation of these genes is associated with mammary tumor development in dogs and women (Uva, Aurisicchio et al. 2009). In human breast cancer, BRCA2 is overexpressed being associated with a poor prognosis whereas the levels of BRCA1 expression decrease during the progression of sporadic breast cancer (Thompson, Jensen et al. 1995; Bieche, Nogues et al. 1999; Maacke, Opitz et al. 2000; Chang and Elledge 2001). Similarly, in canine mammary tumors, the messenger RNA expression of BRCA2 decreases in adenomas and increases in lymph node metastases of mammary adenocarcinomas (Klopfleisch and Gruber 2009), whereas BRCA1 expression decreases, being therefore associated with a malignant phenotype (Nieto, Perez-Alenza et al. 2003).

P53 is a tumor-suppressor gene that plays a central role in rendering the human mammary epithelium resistant to tumorigenesis (Jerry, Dunphy et al. 2010). In canine mammary tumors, P53 gene mutations and protein overexpression are considered a useful predictor of increased malignant potential and poor prognosis (Setoguchi, Sakai et al. 2001; Lee, Kim et al. 2004; Olson 2007; Klopfleisch and Gruber 2009).

P-cadherin and E-cadherin are calcium-dependent cell-cell adhesion molecules with central roles in cancer. P-cadherin is expressed in myoepithelial cells in normal breast tissue and is abnormally overexpressed in high-grade invasive breast carcinomas. The aberrant expression of P-cadherin is associated with poor prognosis in human breast cancer, being reported as an enhancer of cell invasion and tumor aggressiveness (Paredes, Albergaria et al. 2005; Paredes, Correia et al. 2007). In the same way, in canine mammary tumors, it was observed a significant correlation between P-cadherin expression and the histological type (Gama, Paredes et al. 2004), and an association between aberrant P-cadherin expression and the invasive properties of canine malignant mammary tumors (Gama, Paredes et al. 2008). E-cadherin is expressed in epithelial cells playing a critical role in the maintenance of basolateral cell adhesion and polarity,being involved in the normal tissue architecture and homeostasis (van Roy and Berx 2008). In both human breast cancer and canine mammary tumors, the dysfunction or inactivation of E-cadherin is associated with tumor development and progression (Tan, Potts et al. 1999; Matos, Lopes et al. 2006; De Matos, Lopes et al. 2007; Pinho, Matos et al. 2007; Gama, Paredes et al. 2008; Pinho, Reis et al. 2009).

Other molecules with similar roles in both canine and human mammary carcinogenesis are epidermal growth factor receptor (EGFR), estrogen receptors (ERs) and progesterone receptors (PRs) (Chang, Tsai et al. 2009; Gama, Gartner et al. 2009; Pinho 2012).

Glycoscience and Glycomics in Canine: A Model for Human Translational Research

Glycosylation is considered the most diverse and complex form of protein post-translational modification. It is essential for multicellular life and its complete absence is embryonically lethal (Marek, Vijay et al. 1999). Glycosylation is universal to all living forms so that every cell either free-living or part of a multicellular organism has its surface covered with glycans. Moreover, most of the secreted molecules and extracellular matrices of multicellular organisms are rich in glycans and glycoconjugates. Their location on the outer surface of cellular and secreted molecules gives them a privileged position to modulate and mediate a wide variety of events in cell-cell and cell-matrix interactions that are critical to the proper assembly of a complex multicellular organism (Varki 2009).

Glycans (carbohydrates) are one of the four basic components of cells, besides proteins, lipids and nucleic acids, and may also be the most abundant and diverse nature´s biopolymers. Vertebrates, and especially mammals, have evolved a highly complex glycan repertoire that is structurally distinct from that of invertebrates, lower eukaryotes and prokaryotes.

Glycosylation is defined as the enzymatic process that produces glycosidic linkages of saccharides to other saccharides, proteins and lipids. Mammalian glycans are formed by an endogenous portfolio of cellular enzymes and substrates (Helenius and Aebi 2001; Ohtsubo and Marth 2006). The resulting glycome (biological repertoire of glycan structures), particularly the mammalian glycome repertoire is estimated to be between hundreds and thousands of glycans structures containing a significant amount of biological information. Glycans are involved in a myriad of different biological functions that span from those that appear relatively subtle, to those that are crucial to the development, growth, differentiation, or survival of an organism (Varki 1993). They are involved in molecular recognition, inter- and intracellular signaling, embryonic development, fertilization, immune defense, inflammation, cell adhesion and division processes, viral replication, parasitic infections, auto-immune diseases and cancer (Varki 1993). Mammalian glycosylation governs physiology and contributes to disease (Ohtsubo and Marth 2006). Changes in glycosylation are common in many types of diseases with cells frequently displaying glycans at different levels or with fundamental different structures comparing to the normal counterparts (Dube and Bertozzi 2005; Varki 2009).

The glycosylation pattern of eukaryotic cells can therefore be considered as a code for cellular physiology once it is altered with the onset of pathological conditions such as cancer and inflammation (Meezan, Wu et al. 1969; Turner 1992; Mackiewicz and Mackiewicz 1995; Axford 1999; Dube and Bertozzi 2005). Proteins displaying altered glycosylation that are expressed by cancer cells underlies the biomarker detection in the serum of cancer patients (Reis, Osorio et al. 2010).

Concerning canine´s glycome and its role in cellular mechanisms of health and disease, the literature is still poor. Andersson et al, have described a disease-related variations of the glycosylation of haptoglobin in dog. Haptoglobin is a glycoprotein synthesized by the liver that mediates the recycling of heme iron during hemolysis through the formation of a tight complex with hemoglobin that is released by erythrocytes. It was described that some fractions of dog haptoglobin associated with liver disease showed changes in the carbohydrates composition, mainly regarding fucose content (Andersson, Stenstrom et al. 1998). In accordance, it was also reported in human that glycoforms of haptoglobin with altered sialylation and fucosylation are specific to hepatocellular carcinoma being proposed as a biomarker in the diagnosis of hepatocarcinoma (Ang, Poon et al. 2006).

Another report on glycobiology and canine diseases, showed that N-glycans have a role in the pathogenesis of canine distemper virus (Sawatsky and von Messling 2010), which is in accordance with the role of glycans as receptors for virus pathogenesis such as the case of influenza virus in humans, swine and birds (Viswanathan, Chandrasekaran et al. 2010).

In canine tachycardia-induced heart failure studies, it was demonstrated that Calsequestrin glycans in canine heart failure cases had a higher content of mannose residues comparing with normal hearts, suggesting that modifications of the glycosylation of Calsequestrin could be implicated in defective junctional sarcoplasmic reticulum trafficking and $Ca2+$ release complex assembly associated with heart failure (Kiarash, Kelly et al. 2004).

Concerning cancer, changes in glycosylation is considered a universal feature of cancer cells. Aberrant glycosylation expressed in glycoproteins in tumor cells has been implicated as an essential mechanism in defining stage and fate of tumor progression (Hakomori 2002). A family of important molecules related to aberrant glycosylation associated with malignant transformation is sialic acids. Sialic acids are typically found as terminal monosaccharides attached to cell surface glycoproteins and glycolipids. Sialyl Lewis x (sLex) is one of the sialylated carbohydrate antigen that is normally expressed on the surface of human leukocytes (neutrophils, monocytes and some T-lymphocytes) and is involved in the attachment of leukocytes to cytokine-activated endothelial cells through its interaction with the E-selectin cell adhesion molecule, leading to leukocyte extravasation and migration into the tissue, during inflammation (Munro, Lo et al. 1992). Furthermore, the expression of sLex antigen is also increased in several carcinomas being associated with tumor metastases and patients poor prognosis (Kannagi 2004). It was demonstrated that sLex is overexpressed in canine mammary carcinomas comparing with normal mammary mucosa, being associated with increased lymph node metastases (Pinho, Matos et al. 2007). These results demonstrated the importance of sLex in malignant phenotype and tumor progression of canine mammary carcinoma. Furthermore the significant relationship between sLex and lymph node metastases appeal to a practical standpoint because it supports for the first time the use of sLex as a prognostic tumor marker in canine malignant mammary gland tumors (Pinho, Matos et al. 2007). In addition, it was also described the existence of a biologically coordinated relationship between E-cadherin (a classical cell-cell adhesion molecule) and sLex expression. This inverse relationship (termed molecular plasticity) between E-cadherin and the carbohydrate sLex was found to be associated with the process of genesis, dissemination and subsequent metastases in two comparative models: woman inflammatory breast cancer and canine mammary carcinoma (Pinho, Reis et al. 2009).

Another recent report demonstrated that during the acquisition of the malignant phenotype, canine E-cadherin significantly underwent an extensive modification of its glycans composition that was characterized by increased sialylation and increased branching N-glycan structures. These extensive modifications of E-cadherin glycans composition was proposed to be important for the glycoprotein regulation associated with tumor development and progression (Pinho, Osorio et al. 2009).

Another report showed that the transformation of Mardin-Darby Canine Kidney cells (MDCK) by murine sarcoma virus leads to the acquisition of malignant phenotype that was characterized by invasive capacity in vitro and production of invasive and metastatic tumors upon injection into nude mice.

The malignant transformation was shown to be accompanied by changes in the glycosylation of MDCK cells, that was characterized by alterations in sialylation and fucosylation of the cell surface exposed glycans (Bruyneel, Debray et al. 1990).

Another report has shown changes in the glycosylation profile of neoplastic canine endothelial cells. Augustin-Voss et al, demonstrated that during neoplastic transformation there was a phenotypic heterogeneity of the glycans composition of neoplastic endothelial cells comparing with the uniform pattern of glycosylation observed in normal endothelial cells (Augustin-Voss, Smith et al. 1990).

In summary, glycosylation is an appealing and emerging molecular mechanism underlying mammalian homeostasis and pathologies. In fact, genomics and proteomics have produced unparalleled discoveries that have advanced the understanding of biological processes, however the picture is incomplete. We believe that the next level of discoveries that may help treat and cure diseases will be glycomics (study of carbohydrates and its role in biology). There are compelling evidences, as demonstrated above, that studying canine´s glycome is an attractive way of understanding fundamental biological processes such as cancer, as a model for human carcinogenesis.

From Canine to Human Cancer: An Opportunity for New Cancer Treatments

Dogs with cancer are considered a promising tool in clinical trials. Clinical studies using dogs as pre-clinical models have great benefits for the development and testing of new cancer drugs: the large body size of canines facilitates the collection of biologic samples (serum, urine and serial tissue biopsy), the homology of hepatic enzyme and the same cancer-associated molecular targets of dogs and humans are some of the advantages of using dogs as pre-clinical models. The integration of pet dogs in clinical trials provides an opportunity to assess safety and activity of a novel drug and evaluate efficacy, pharmacokinetics/dynamics, toxicity, dosing, biomarkers/endpoints, and adverse effects of new drugs before the first in-human studies (Paoloni and Khanna 2008; Rowell, McCarthy et al. 2011).

Several studies in comparative oncology have been developed to evaluate novel therapeutics strategies for a variety of cancers. Recently, a phase I clinical trial using dogs with spontaneous cancers has characterized the toxicity and biologic effective doses of a potential new agent with antitumor activity, PEGylated-tumor necrosis factor-α (PEGylated-TNFα), supporting its clinical evaluation in human cancers (Thamm, Kurzman et al. 2010).

An additional phase I clinical study has assessed pharmacokinetics, toxicity, and tumor responses to SU11654, an indolinone receptor tyrosine kinase (RTK) inhibitor. RTKs are involved in the control of cellular proliferation, and their aberrant signaling in cancer context makes them an important target for the development of anticancer therapies. This preclinical study in dogs showed that SU11654 exhibited activity against a variety of spontaneous tumors in canine models, giving evidence of similar biologic responses in human cancers (Ullrich and Schlessinger 1990; Griffin 2001; London, Hannah et al. 2003).

Conclusion

Taking into consideration the close similarity of canine and human biology at genomics, proteomics and glycomics levels, it is plausible to consider canine tumors as a valuable and powerful model for studying such a complex biological system that is cancer. This comparative oncology approach will certainly contribute to benefit both species.

References

Alison, M. R. (2004). The Cancer Handbook, John Wiley and Sons.

Andersson, M., M. Stenstrom, et al. (1998). "Disease-related variations of the glycosylation of haptoglobin in the dog." *J. Comp. Pathol.* 119(3): 227-238.

Ang, I. L., T. C. Poon, et al. (2006). "Study of serum haptoglobin and its glycoforms in the diagnosis of hepatocellular carcinoma: a glycoproteomic approach." *J. Proteome Res.* 5(10): 2691-2700.

Augustin-Voss, H. G., C. A. Smith, et al. (1990). "Phenotypic characterization of normal and neoplastic canine endothelial cells by lectin histochemistry." *Vet. Pathol.* 27(2): 103-109.

Axford, J. S. (1999). "Glycosylation and rheumatic disease." *Biochim. Biophys. Acta.* 1455(2-3): 219-229.

Becher, O. J. and E. C. Holland (2006). "Genetically engineered models have advantages over xenografts for preclinical studies." *Cancer Res.* 66(7): 3355-3358, discussion 3358-3359.

Bieche, I., C. Nogues, et al. (1999). "Overexpression of BRCA2 gene in sporadic breast tumors." *Oncogene* 18(37): 5232-5238.

Bruyneel, E. A., H. Debray, et al. (1990). "Altered glycosylation in Madin-Darby canine kidney (MDCK) cells after transformation by murine sarcoma virus." *Clin. Exp. Metastasis* 8(3): 241-253.

Castaneda, C. A., H. Cortes-Funes, et al. (2010). "The phosphatidyl inositol 3-kinase/AKT signaling pathway in breast cancer." *Cancer Metastasis Rev.* 29(4): 751-759.

Cespedes, M. V., I. Casanova, et al. (2006). "Mouse models in oncogenesis and cancer therapy." *Clin. Transl. Oncol.* 8(5): 318-329.

Chang, C. C., M. H. Tsai, et al. (2009). "Evaluation of hormone receptor expression for use in predicting survival of female dogs with malignant mammary gland tumors." *J. Am. Vet. Med. Assoc.* 235(4): 391-396.

Chang, J. and R. M. Elledge (2001). "Clinical management of women with genomic BRCA1 and BRCA2 mutations." *Breast Cancer Res. Treat* 69(2): 101-113.

De Matos, A. J., C. C. Lopes, et al. (2007). "E-cadherin, beta-catenin, invasion and lymph node metastases in canine malignant mammary tumors." *APMIS* 115(4): 327-334.

De Vico, G., P. Maiolino, et al. (2005). "Spontaneous tumors of pet dog as models for human cancers: searching for adequate guidelines." *Riv. Biol.* 98(2): 279-296.

Dillon, R. L., D. E. White, et al. (2007). "The phosphatidyl inositol 3-kinase signaling network: implications for human breast cancer." *Oncogene* 26(9): 1338-1345.

Dube, D. H. and C. R. Bertozzi (2005). "Glycans in cancer and inflammation--potential for therapeutics and diagnostics." *Nat. Rev. Drug Discov.* 4(6): 477-488.

Galanis, A., A. Pappa, et al. (2008). "Reactive oxygen species and HIF-1 signalling in cancer." *Cancer Lett.* 266(1): 12-20.

Gama, A., F. Gartner, et al. (2009). "Immunohistochemical expression of Epidermal Growth Factor Receptor (EGFR) in canine mammary tissues." *Res. Vet. Sci.* 87(3): 432-437.

Gama, A., J. Paredes, et al. (2004). "P-cadherin expression in canine mammary tissues." *J. Comp. Pathol.* 130(1): 13-20.

Gama, A., J. Paredes, et al. (2008). "Expression of E-cadherin, P-cadherin and beta-catenin in canine malignant mammary tumors in relation to clinicopathological parameters, proliferation and survival." *Vet. J.* 177(1): 45-53.

Gordon, I. K. and C. Khanna (2010). "Modeling opportunities in comparative oncology for drug development." *ILAR J.* 51(3): 214-220.

Griffin, J. (2001). "The biology of signal transduction inhibition: basic science to novel therapies." *Semin. Oncol.* 28(5 Suppl 17): 3-8.

Hakomori, S. (2002). "Glycosylation defining cancer malignancy: new wine in an old bottle." *Proc. Natl. Acad. Sci.* U S A 99(16): 10231-10233.

Hanahan, D. and R. A. Weinberg (2011). "Hallmarks of cancer: the next generation." *Cell* 144(5): 646-674.

Hansen, K. and C. Khanna (2004). "Spontaneous and genetically engineered animal models; use in preclinical cancer drug development." *Eur. J. Cancer* 40(6): 858-880.

Helenius, A. and M. Aebi (2001). "Intracellular functions of N-linked glycans." *Science* 291(5512): 2364-2369.

Jerry, D. J., K. A. Dunphy, et al. (2010). "Estrogens, regulation of p53 and breast cancer risk: a balancing act." *Cell Mol. Life Sci.* 67(7): 1017-1023.

Kannagi, R. (2004). "Molecular mechanism for cancer-associated induction of sialyl Lewis X and sialyl Lewis A expression-The Warburg effect revisited." *Glycoconj. J.* 20(5): 353-364.

Kiarash, A., C. E. Kelly, et al. (2004). "Defective glycosylation of calsequestrin in heart failure." *Cardiovasc. Res.* 63(2): 264-272.

Klopfleisch, R. and A. D. Gruber (2009). "Increased Expression of BRCA2 and RAD51 in Lymph Node Metastases of Canine Mammary Adenocarcinomas." *Veterinary Pathology* 46(3): 416-422.

Klopfleisch, R., H. von Euler, et al. (2011). "Molecular carcinogenesis of canine mammary tumors: news from an old disease." *Vet. Pathol.* 48(1): 98-116.

Knapp, D. W. and D. J. Waters (1997). "Naturally occurring cancer in pet dogs: important models for developing improved cancer therapy for humans." *Mol. Med. Today* 3(1): 8-11.

Lee, C. H., W. H. Kim, et al. (2004). "Mutation and overexpression of p53 as a prognostic factor in canine mammary tumors." *J. Vet. Sci.* 5(1): 63-69.

London, C. A., A. L. Hannah, et al. (2003). "Phase I dose-escalating study of SU11654, a small molecule receptor tyrosine kinase inhibitor, in dogs with spontaneous malignancies." *Clin. Cancer Res.* 9(7): 2755-2768.

Maacke, H., S. Opitz, et al. (2000). "Over-expression of wild-type Rad51 correlates with histological grading of invasive ductal breast cancer." *Int. J. Cancer*. 88(6): 907-913.

MacEwen, E. G. (1990). "Spontaneous tumors in dogs and cats: models for the study of cancer biology and treatment." *Cancer Metastasis Rev.* 9(2): 125-136.

Mackiewicz, A. and K. Mackiewicz (1995). "Glycoforms of serum alpha 1-acid glycoprotein as markers of inflammation and cancer." *Glycoconj. J.* 12(3): 241-247.

Marek, K. W., I. K. Vijay, et al. (1999). "A recessive deletion in the GlcNAc-1-phosphotransferase gene results in peri-implantation embryonic lethality." *Glycobiology* 9(11): 1263-1271.

Masters, J. R. (2002). "HeLa cells 50 years on: the good, the bad and the ugly." *Nat. Rev. Cancer* 2(4): 315-319.

Matos, A. J., C. Lopes, et al. (2006). "E-cadherin expression in canine malignant mammary tumors: relationship to other clinico-pathological variables." *J. Comp. Pathol.* 134(2-3): 182-189.

Meezan, E., H. C. Wu, et al. (1969). "Comparative studies on the carbohydrate-containing membrane components of normal and virus-transformed mouse fibroblasts. II. Separation of glycoproteins and glycopeptides by sephadex chromatography." *Biochemistry* 8(6): 2518-2524.

Milovanovic, Z., R. Dzodic, et al. (2011). "PTEN protein expression in postmenopausal steroid receptor positive early breast cancer patients treated with adjuvant tamoxifen." *J. BUON* 16(1): 46-51.

Munro, J. M., S. K. Lo, et al. (1992). "Expression of sialyl-Lewis X, an E-selectin ligand, in inflammation, immune processes, and lymphoid tissues." *Am. J. Pathol.* 141(6): 1397-1408.

Nieto, A., M. D. Perez-Alenza, et al. (2003). "BRCA1 expression in canine mammary dysplasias and tumors: relationship with prognostic variables." *J. Comp. Pathol.* 128(4): 260-268.

Ohtsubo, K. and J. D. Marth (2006). "Glycosylation in cellular mechanisms of health and disease." *Cell* 126(5): 855-867.

Olson, P. N. (2007). "Using the canine genome to cure cancer and other diseases." *Theriogenology*. 68(3): 378-381.

Paoloni, M. and C. Khanna (2008). "Translation of new cancer treatments from pet dogs to humans." *Nat. Rev. Cancer* 8(2): 147-156.

Paredes, J., A. Albergaria, et al. (2005). "P-cadherin overexpression is an indicator of clinical outcome in invasive breast carcinomas and is associated with CDH3 promoter hypomethylation." *Clinical Cancer Research* 11(16): 5869-5877.

Paredes, J., A. L. Correia, et al. (2007). "P-cadherin expression in breast cancer: a review." *Breast Cancer Res.* 9(5): 214.

Pinho, S. S., Carvalho, S., Cabral, J., Reis, C.A., Gärtner, F. (2012). *"Canine tumors: a spontaneous animal model of human carcinogenesis."* Translational Research in press.

Pinho, S. S., A. J. Matos, et al. (2007). "Sialyl Lewis x expression in canine malignant mammary tumors: correlation with clinicopathological features and E-Cadherin expression." *BMC Cancer* 7: 124.

Pinho, S. S., H. Osorio, et al. (2009). "Role of E-cadherin N-glycosylation profile in a mammary tumor model." *Biochem. Biophys. Res. Commun.* 379(4): 1091-1096.

Pinho, S. S., C. A. Reis, et al. (2009). "Molecular plasticity of E-cadherin and sialyl lewis x expression, in two comparative models of mammary tumorigenesis." *PLoS One* 4(8): e6636.

Rangarajan, A. and R. A. Weinberg (2003). "Opinion: Comparative biology of mouse versus human cells: modelling human cancer in mice." Nat. *Rev. Cancer* 3(12): 952-959.

Reis, C. A., H. Osorio, et al. (2010). "Alterations in glycosylation as biomarkers for cancer detection." *J. Clin. Pathol.* 63(4): 322-329.

Ressel, L., F. Millanta, et al. (2009). "Reduced PTEN protein expression and its prognostic implications in canine and feline mammary tumors." *Vet. Pathol.* 46(5): 860-868.

Richmond, A. and Y. Su (2008). "Mouse xenograft models vs GEM models for human cancer therapeutics." *Dis. Model Mech.* 1(2-3): 78-82.

Rowell, J. L., D. O. McCarthy, et al. (2011). "Dog models of naturally occurring cancer." *Trends Mol. Med.* 17(7): 380-388.

Saal, L. H., P. Johansson, et al. (2007). "Poor prognosis in carcinoma is associated with a gene expression signature of aberrant PTEN tumor suppressor pathway activity." *Proc. Natl. Acad. Sci. U S A.* 104(18): 7564-7569.

Sawatsky, B. and V. von Messling (2010). "Canine distemper viruses expressing a hemagglutinin without N-glycans lose virulence but retain immunosuppression." *J. Virol.* 84(6): 2753-2761.

Sebolt-Leopold, J. S. and R. Herrera (2004). "Targeting the mitogen-activated protein kinase cascade to treat cancer." *Nat. Rev. Cancer* 4(12): 937-947.

Setoguchi, A., T. Sakai, et al. (2001). "Aberrations of the p53 tumor suppressor gene in various tumors in dogs." *Am. J. Vet. Res.* 62(3): 433-439.

Singh, G., L. Odriozola, et al. (2011). "Characterization of a novel PTEN mutation in MDA-MB-453 breast carcinoma cell line." *BMC Cancer* 11: 490.

Sweet-Cordero, A., S. Mukherjee, et al. (2005). "An oncogenic KRAS2 expression signature identified by cross-species gene-expression analysis." *Nat. Genet* 37(1): 48-55.

Tan, D. S. P., H. W. W. Potts, et al. (1999). "The biological and prognostic significance of cell polarity and E-cadherin in grade I infiltrating ductal carcinoma of the breast." *Journal of Pathology* 189(1): 20-27.

Teicher, B. A. (2009). "In vivo/ex vivo and in situ assays used in cancer research: a brief review." *Toxicol. Pathol.* 37(1): 114-122.

Thamm, D. H., I. D. Kurzman, et al. (2010). "Preclinical investigation of PEGylated tumor necrosis factor alpha in dogs with spontaneous tumors: phase I evaluation." *Clin. Cancer Res.* 16(5): 1498-1508.

Thompson, M. E., R. A. Jensen, et al. (1995). "Decreased expression of BRCA1 accelerates growth and is often present during sporadic breast cancer progression." *Nat. Genet.* 9(4): 444-450.

Turner, G. A. (1992). "N-glycosylation of serum proteins in disease and its investigation using lectins." *Clin. Chim. Acta.* 208(3): 149-171.

Ullrich, A. and J. Schlessinger (1990). "Signal transduction by receptors with tyrosine kinase activity." *Cell* 61(2): 203-212.

Uva, P., L. Aurisicchio, et al. (2009). "Comparative expression pathway analysis of human and canine mammary tumors." *BMC Genomics* 10: 135.

Vail, D. M. and E. G. MacEwen (2000). "Spontaneously occurring tumors of companion animals as models for human cancer." *Cancer Invest.* 18(8): 781-792.

van Roy, F. and G. Berx (2008). "The cell-cell adhesion molecule E-cadherin." *Cellular and Molecular Life Sciences* 65(23): 3756-3788.

Varki, A. (1993). "Biological Roles of Oligosaccharides - All of the Theories Are Correct." *Glycobiology* 3(2): 97-130.

Varki, A. (1993). "Biological roles of oligosaccharides: all of the theories are correct." *Glycobiology* 3(2): 97-130.

Varki, A. (2009). Essentials of glycobiology. Cold Spring Harbor New York, Cold Spring Harbor Laboratory Press.

Venkitaraman, A. R. (2002). "Cancer susceptibility and the functions of BRCA1 and BRCA2." *Cell* 108(2): 171-182.

Viswanathan, K., A. Chandrasekaran, et al. (2010). "Glycans as receptors for influenza pathogenesis." *Glycoconj. J.* 27(6): 561-570.

Voskoglou-Nomikos, T., J. L. Pater, et al. (2003). "Clinical predictive value of the in vitro cell line, human xenograft, and mouse allograft preclinical cancer models." *Clinical Cancer Research* 9(11): 4227-4239.

In: Canine Behavior, Classification and Diseases ISBN: 978-1-62081-304-1
Editors: R. L. Andrade and C. I. Batista

Chapter IV

Important Parasitic Zoonosis in Dogs

Katia Denise Saraiva Bresciani, Willian Marinho Dourado Coelho, Juliana de Carvalho Apolinário Coelho, Natalia Marinho Dourado Coelho, Milena Araúz Viol, Jancarlo Ferreira Gomes and Alvimar José da Costa

Departamento de Apoio, Produção e Saúde Animal, Faculdade de Odontologia de Araçatuba - FOA, Universidade do Estado de São Paulo - UNESP, Araçatuba - SP, Brazil

Abstract

The dog can be involved in the mechanical transmission of infection by helminthes and protozoa; it has an epidemiological role in these zoonoses. The high rate of dogs naturally infected by endoparasites and the great possibility of acquiring this parasite justify the importance of attempting to prevent the occurrence of this illness. The aim of this paper is to demonstrate, through literature review, some clinical, epidemic and pathological aspects of endoparasite infection in the canine species.

Introduction

Dogs play a relevant role as definitive hosts of a large number of endoparasites, shedding gastrointestinal helminth larvae and eggs and protozoan cysts and oocysts in their feces, which favors environmental contamination and possible spread of diseases.

Considering the close proximity between men and pets, determining the occurrence of endoparasites in small animals has become increasingly relevant. These diseases are frequently diagnosed in spite of the existent therapeutic and prophylactic measures.

Protozoal Infections

Toxoplasmosis

Infection by *Toxoplasma gondii* is particularly interesting from the point of view of public health. Although generally asymptomatic, it frequently shows severe clinical signs of reactivation or fatal outcomes in immunosuppressed patients. Behavioral changes such as attention deficit, schizophrenia, obsessive compulsive disorder, epilepsy and hyperactivity have been reported (Lafferty, 2005, Pradhan et al., 2007, Prandota, 2010).

Women in initial stages of gestation may undergo miscarriage, premature birth, neonatal death and even the classical Sabin's Triad, characterized by retinochoroiditis, cerebral calcifications, hydrocephaly or microcephaly (Jones et al., 2001, Soares et al., 2011).

Surveys of toxoplasmosis are essential for production animals and pets. Reproductive disorders were already proved in several species, including men and dogs, emphasizing the relevance of studies of congenital toxoplasmosis and its reflexes (Bresciani et al., 1999, Bresciani et al., 2001, Bresciani et al., 2009, Azevedo et al., 2010).

In its cycle, *T. gondii* shows itself as two evolutionary forms: tachyzoites, present in organic liquid in the acute phase, and tissue cysts in the chronic infection. On the other hand, oocysts are the final product of sexual reproduction and are only formed in the digestive tract of felids, definitive hosts which release oocysts together with their feces, where, through sporogony, the oocysts become infective and extremely resistant to the environmental conditions (Miller et al., 1972).

The protozoan can be transmitted especially by ingestion of tissue cysts present in raw or undercooked meat, by contamination of food with oocysts from the feces of infected felids and by transplacental route. Other less important forms are ingestion of contaminated milk, organic fluid transference and organ transplantation (Dubey, 2009).

Some dogs remain asymptomatic, a few become sick and deaths are rare (Dubey, 1985). However, pulmonary and digestive disorders (Oppermann, 1971), hyperthermia, lymphadenopathy (Bresciani et al., 2001), ocular lesions (Abreu et al., 2002) and neuropathies (Brito et al., 2002) may occur.

Detection of antibodies against *T. gondii* can be done by indirect immunofluorescence reaction, as well as by modified agglutination test, hemagglutination test and Enzyme Linked Immunosorbent Assay (ELISA).

We observed miscarriage, fetal and neonatal mortality in pregnant dogs and detected the parasite in saliva, milk and urine of infected mothers of serologically positive but apparently healthy pups (Bresciani et al., 2009). It is also important to note that we further confirmed sexual transmission (Arantes et al., 2009).

Toxoplasmosis seroprevalence is high in the canine species and increases with age, especially in stray ones (Souza et al., 2003, Cañón-Franco et al., 2004), which contribute to the mechanical spread of this disease (Frenkel and Parker, 1996; Lindsay et al.,1997, Schares et al., 2005).

Some drugs such as pyrimethamine, trimethoprim associated with sulfonamide and doxycycline, doxycycline, azithromycin, minocycline, clarithromycin and clindamycin can be employed (Greene, 1990; Lappin, 2004).

Thus, coprophagy must be prevented, while the supply of cooked meat products or commercial food is recommended. We verified higher incidence of infection by *T. gondii* among dogs kept on earth or grass ground (Bresciani et al., 2007) and isolated oocysts of this parasite from sand from parks in public schools with potential risk of contamination for children (Santos et al., 2010).

Canine Visceral Leishmaniosis or Calazar

Showing cosmopolitan distribution, enzootic infections caused by morphologically similar protozoa of the genus *Leishmania* (Monteiro et al., 2005, Lindoso and Goto, 2006) can be transmitted by sand flies (Brasil, 2006).

Leishmaniasis is considered by the World Health Organization (WHO) the second most important current protozoal infection in people. Human patients subjected to chemotherapy are also more susceptible and, without treatment, the disease is lethal in 95% cases (Brasil, 2006). Estimates indicate that 16 to 18 millions are affected in the world (Rosypal et al., 2007).

In humans, the signs of infection by *Leishmania* spp. are generally auto-limiting and subclinical and may progress to fever, cachexia, hepatosplenomegaly, copious bleeding and even death.

The sand fly(like *Lutzomyia* spp.) becomes infected while ingesting, during blood feeding, amastigote forms of the parasite, present in the cells of the monocytic phagocyte system on the dermis of the infected host. In the digestive tube of the insect, amastigotes change into promastigotes. During a new blood feeding, the female of the infected insect inoculate these infective forms into the definitive host where they undergo phagocytosis by macrophages, returning to amastigote form and multiplying to cause cell rupture. Thus, there is hematogenic dissemination to tissues like liver, spleen, lymph node and bone marrow (Lainson and Shaw, 1987).

Some dogs manifest a few clinical signs such as rare cutaneous lesions and nodules, while others become cachectic, showing ophthalmologic changes, onychogryphosis, and dermatopathies like peeling, nodules and ulcers, especially in the edges of ears or spread all over the body. Cases of paresis of the hind limbs have been described, as well as increased volume of the spleen and lymph nodes, including diarrhea (Silva et al., 2001).

We studied cross infections by *Leishmania* spp. and *Trypanossoma* spp. using Indirect Immunoenzyme Assay (ELISA), Indirect Fluorescent Antibody Test (IFAT) and Polymerase Chain Reaction (PCR) and we observed cross infections by both protozoa in the animals analyzed in this study.

The treatment of canine visceral leishmaniasis, for unknown reasons, is more complicated than that of humans and no medicine is totally efficient in eliminating this parasitic infection, remaining the risk of recurrence after therapy. In endemic regions, a drug protocol consists in the association between allopurinol and pentavalent antimonial like meglumine.

Several immunogens have been tested, including live or inactivated vaccines, purified fractions of Leishmania, recombinant antigens, antigen expression and *Leishmania* plasmid DNA through the recombinant bacterium (Lima et al., 2010).

The fox is the main reservoir of this disease in the wild and rural environment, while the dog plays this role in the urban environment (São Paulo, 2006). The Brazilian Ministry of Health recommends euthanasia for affected animals (BRASIL, 2006, Troncarelli, 2008).

This reemerging illness has characterized an epidemiological transition process, with increasing incidence and geographic expansion in urban areas previously free from this problem (Alves and Bevilacqua, 2004).

This canine disease, has preceded the occurrence of human cases (Paranhos-Silva et al., 1996) and is associated with environments of low socio-economic level (Alves and Bevilacqua, 2004, BrasiL, 2006), showing high seroprevalence and lethality in endemic areas (Silva et al., 2001, Bepa, 2010).

Cryptosporidiosis

By means of molecular characterization, 20 species are established for the genus *Cryptosporidium* (Plutzer and Karanis, 2009, Fayer, 2010); dogs are commonly infected by *C. parvum* (Xiao et al., 1999) and *C. canis* (Thomaz et al., 2007), while humans are frequently affected by *C. parvum* and *C. hominis* (Fayer et al., 2001, Smith et al., 2009).

Cryptosporidium protozoa are included in the Neglected Diseases Initiative of the WHO due to their close relationship with deficient sanitation and low income of the population; thus, they are considered responsible for child malnutrition, organic deficit and death. For immunocompetent ones, the infection does not manifest clinically in communities from endemic areas or causes auto-limiting diarrhea with abdominal pain and vomits (Thompson et al., 2008).

In its biology, *Cryptosporidium* sporulated oocysts are ingested by the host and, following exposure to the gastric juice and pancreatic enzymes, excystation occurs in the duodenum, releasing four sporozoites. The latter are involved by microvilli and are located in a parasitophorous vacuole, starting the asexual reproduction (merogony). The four merozoites released in the second merogony originate the sexual stages, microgametes and macrogametes; the latter unit to form the zygote, which after two divisions forms the oocyst. Sporulation occurs inside the oocyst, developing four sporozoites. Thus, thin-walled oocysts (capable of starting a new cycle inside the same host) and thick-walled oocysts are formed and released to the outer environment together with the fecal content. The infection generally remains in the gastrointestinal tract (Tzipori and Griffths, 1998, Thompson et al., 2008).

Diarrhea due to malabsorption is caused by epithelial barrier rupture and immunological and inflammatory responses of the host. Infection by *Cryptosporidium* causes atrophy, fusion and inflammation on the surface of intestinal microvilli, which result in absorptive surface loss and unbalanced nutrient transport (Thompson et al., 2008).

Asymptomatic signs, with release of a few fecal oocysts, can be commonly detected in dogs (Thompson et al., 2008). All over the world, variable prevalence of this infection (from complete absence to rates of 44.1%) has been reported, showing higher occurrence in the young and relationship to weaning, nutritional deficiencies and agglomeration in kennels (Hammes et al., 2007, Mundim et al., 2007, Lallo and Bondan, 2006, Bresciani et al., 2008).

We observed these evolutionary forms by techniques that stain the oocysts, such as Malachite green, Ziehl-Nielsen and Kinyoun. In a study performed by our team, the parasitological tests of Kinyoun and Sheather were compared with ELISA and the latter was more sensitive in detecting infection by *Cryptosporidium* spp. in dogs (Bresciani et al., 2008).

The distinction between *Cryptoporidium* species and genotypes has been conclusive only by molecular characterization. In spite of scientific advances, these cytogenetic analyses are costly and thus maintain the interest in searching for diagnostic methods that can be performed by veterinarians to confirm the clinical suspect and to adopt immediate therapeutic measures (Plutzer and Karanis, 2009).

Nitazoxanide minimized diarrhea and oocyst release and is the first drug approved for the treatment of cryptosporidiosis (Rossignol., 2010).

Considering the disease control, our research group interviewed 188 guardians of children with the aim of verifying the degree of contact between the child and respective pet.

A total of 55.9% (104/186) parents confirmed that the animals lick the face of their children, 73.6% (137/186) pets enter the bedroom, 11.2% (21/186) pets jump and/or sleep on the bed with the children, only 7.5% (14/186) children wash their hands after having played with the animal, and 54.8% children (102/186) play with sand at home. Of the four children positive for *Cryptosporidium* spp. according to ELISA, three had their animals reactive (Coelho, 2009).

Although the risk of infection for men by direct or indirect contact with small animals is not determined (Fayer et al., 2001, Smith et al., 2009), the fecal oocysts released by dogs may represent a source of human infection and are rarely resistant to the environmental conditions (Plutzer and Karanis, 2009)

Helminthiasis

Visceral Larva Migrans Syndrome (Beaver et al., 1952) can be caused by *Toxocara canis* and Cutaneous Larva Migrans Syndrome by *A. caninum* or *A. braziliense* (Lee, 1874) in humans.

The high frequency of *Ancylostoma* spp. and *T. canis* justifies the concern about this worldwide problem, emphasizing its relevance from an epidemic-sanitary point of view (Táparo et al., 2006), since evolutionary forms of helminthes released in the fecal content of dogs lead to high environmental contamination (Brener et al., 2005, Pfukenyi et al., 2010).

Visceral Larva Migrans (VLM)

VLM is a cosmopolitan anthropozoonosis. Serological surveys have confirmed the dissemination of *T. canis* among the human population (Chieffi and Müller, 1976). The contact with the soil, fomites or hands contaminated by the feces of animals infected with these agents may lead to accidental transmission to people (Blazius, 2006).

Human infection by *T. canis* occurs by the ingestion of larval eggs present in the soil or hands contaminated with the feces of infected animals. The parasite does not reach maturity in these hosts, but the larvae remain alive, erratically migrating in internal organs and producing a pathology named Visceral Larva Migrans (VLM) or invading the ocular globe and causing Ocular Larva Migrans (OLM).

In toxocariasis, asymptomatic signs are evidenced, as well as fever, hypereosinophilia, hepatomegaly, ocular, pulmonary or cardiac manifestations, nephrosis and signs of cerebral lesion in humans (Overgaauw, 1997).

The enterohepatic pneumoenteral form is considered the most common infection form in dogs aged up to three months. Above such age range, this migration type occurred at a lower frequency. In pregnant dogs, migrating larvae mobilize at approximately three weeks before parturition and migrate to the fetal lungs, molting to third-instar larvae before birth. In the newborn pup, the cycle is completed when the larva migrates through the trachea and to the intestinal lumen, where molts to adult worms finally occur (Urquhart, 1991).

As regards pathogenic lesions caused by gastrointestinal parasites, we must consider cutaneous, pulmonary (by pulmonary migration of the larva during its development) and intestinal changes due to the final location of the worm in the adult stage (Fortes, 2004).

In dogs, these helminthiases may lead to organic unbalance such as anemia, changes in the appetite, intestinal obstruction or perforation, limited assimilation of nutrients, diarrhea, apathy and sometimes death (Fortes, 2004).

We found high occurrence of *T. canis* (67.3%) in young dogs. Infections by this helminth are more frequent until the age of one year (Gennari et al., 2001). Although adults tend to show effective immune response against ascarids, post-parturition females can release eggs of *Toxocara* spp. in their fecal content (Urquhart et al. 1991).

The latter are known for their resistance to environmental adversities, remaining viable for many years depending on the type of climate and soil (Glickman and Schantz, 1981). In the laboratorial routine, we examine fecal samples from dogs in their first year of life containing a marked quantity of *T. canis* eggs.

Cutaneous Larva Migrans (CLM)

CLM has worldwide importance and is characterized by a parasitic dermatitis caused by the penetration and the migration of larvae of some species of Ancylostomatidae with zoonotic potential into the epithelial extract of the human skin (Broker et al, 2004, Vasconcellos et al., 2006).

Two parasites of small animals are the main etiologic agents of eosinophilic enteritis (Landmann and Prociv, 2003) and cutaneous larva migrans (Caumes, 2006): *Ancylostoma caninum*, with worldwide distribution, and *Ancylostoma braziliense,* especially evidenced in tropical and subtropical regions of the world (Hoff et al., 2008).

Reports of cutaneous larva migrans have been related to children in strict contact with sand from recreation areas, public squares, clubs and child day care centers (Santarém et al., 2004, Moro et al., 2008), as well as to adults who act in contact with the soil such as gardeners, farmers and miners (Hoff et al., 2008). It is common in poor regions of developing countries and sometimes described in places of high purchasing power like tourism areas which are endemic for this disease (Helkelbach and Jackson, 2008).

The man becomes infected by the percutaneous route and *Ancylostoma* larvae start the dermal migration, producing "inflammatory tunnels" which evidence the helminth path on the skin surface. These lesions are generally seen in the regions of feet, legs and buttocks, which become particularly exposed in barefoot individuals or those sitting on the sand. Irritability, insomnia, intense skin pruritus and secondary bacterial infections also constitute frequent symptoms (Helkelbach et al., 2007, Hoff et al., 2008).

This hematophagous nematode of the small intestine of dogs causes acute or chronic hemorrhagic anemia followed by diarrhea which may contain blood and mucus. Its main form of transmission is by the translactational route. Young animals are most frequently affected, but this infection may occur in dogs of all ages by the percutaneous route or by the ingestion of larvae together with food and water (Urquhart et al., 1996, Boag et al, 2003; Blazius et al 2005, Táparo et al., 2006).

Ancylostomatidae can be identified by means of different parasitological techniques, reaching occurrence of 70% to 95.6% (Yacob et al., 2007, Coelho et al., 2011). We evidenced 64.2% (27/42) positivity for *Ancylostoma* in samples collected from the environment. Of this sampling, 10.86% (5/46) were from child day care centers/parks, 41.30% (19/46) from streets/sidewalks and 47.82% (22/46) from squares/gardens (Coelho et al., 2011).

We observed that the methods Willis-Mollay and Sedimentation is considered superior, compared to the Direct method and zinc sulfate flotation centrifugation, to detect these evolutionary and parasitic forms (Taparo et al., 2006).

Parasitological necropsy is considered the gold standard test to elucidate clinical suspicions, either in tests of anthelmintic efficacy or in comparisons between diagnosis techniques for helminth infections (Ogassawara et al., 1986).

Based on the high occurrence of hookworm in dogs and cats in our studies, treatment with anthelmintics is needed, even for animals with negative stool tests, besides adopting a control of the number of animals in public places in order to decrease the likelihood of environmental contamination, since this parasite represents a potential hazard to human and animal health.

Thus, with our scientific studies, we proved that the owners are greatly misinformed about the control of the parasitic diseases mentioned here and about responsible pet ownership, evidencing the need of continuous implantation of community awareness campaigns (Tome et al., 2005, Neto et al., 2011).

References

Abreu, CB.; Navarro, IT.; Reis, ACF.; Souza, MSB.; Machado, R.; Marana, ERM.; Prudêncio, LB.; Mattos, MR.; Tsutsui, VS. 2002. Toxoplasmose ocular em cães jovens inoculados com *Toxoplasma gondii*. *Ciência Rural*, Santa Maria. Vol. 32, Nº 5, 2002, pp.807-812, 0103-8478.

Alves, WA.; Bevilacqua, PD. 2004. Reflexões sobre a qualidade do diagnóstico da leishmaniose visceral canina em inquéritos epidemiológicos: o caso da epidemia de Belo Horizonte, Mina Gerais, Brasil, 1993-1997. *Cadernos de Saúde Pública*, Vol. 20, Nº.1, 2004, pp. 259-265, 1678-4464.

Arantes, TP.; Lopes, WDZ.; Ferreira, RM.; Pieroni, JS.; Pinto, VMR.; Sakamoto, CA.; Costa, AJ. 2009. Toxoplasma gondii: Evidence for the transmission by semen in dogs *Experimental Parasitology*, Vol. 123, Nº. 2, october 2009, pp. 190–194, 0014-4894.

Azevedo, KM.; Setúbal, S.; Lopes, VGS.; Camacho, LAB.; Oliveira, SA. 2010. Congenital toxoplasmosis transmitted by human immunodeficiency-virus infected women. *The Brazilian Journal of Infectious Diseases*. Vol.14, Nº.2, March-April 2010, pp.186-189, 1413-8670.

Beaver, PC.;, Syndrer, CH.; Carrera, GM.; Dent, JH.; Lafferty, JW. 1952. Chronic eosinophilia due to visceral larva migrans: report of three cases. *Pediatrics*. Vol. 9, Nº. 1, january 1952, pp. 7-9, 08739781.

Bepa Comite de leishmaniose visceral americana (2010). Classificação epidemiológica dos municípios segundo o programa de vigilância e controle da leishmaniose visceral americana no estado de São Paulo, atualizado em maio de 2010. *Boletim Epidemiologico Paulista*. Vol. 7, 2010, pp.21-40, 1806-4272.

Blazius, RD.; Emerick, S.; Prophiro, JS.; Romao, PRT.; Silva, OS. 2005. Ocorrência de protozoários e helmintos em amostras de fezes de cães errantes da cidade de Itapema, Santa Catarina. *Revista da Sociedade Brasileira de Medicina Tropical*. Vol. 38, Nº. 1, jan./feb. 2005, pp. 73-74, 0037-8682.

Blazius, RD.; Silva, OS.; Kauling, AL.; Rodrigues, DFP.; Lima, MC. 2006. Contaminação da areia do balneário de Laguna, SC, por Ancylostoma spp. e Toxocara spp. em amostras fecais de cães e gatos. *Arquivo Catarinense de Medicina*. Vol. 35, pp. 55-58.

Boag PR.; Parsons, JC.; Presidente, PJ.; Spithill, TW.; Sexton, JL. 2003 Characterization of humoral immune responses in dogs vaccinated with irradiated *Ancylostoma caninum*. *Veterinary Immunology and Immunopathology*. Vol. 92, Nº.1-2, march 2003, pp. 87-94, 0165-2427.

Brasil. Ministério da Saúde. Secretaria de Vigilância em Saúde. Departamento de Vigilância Epidemiológica. *Manual de Vigilância e Controle da Leishmaniose Visceral*. Brasília, 2006. pp. 9-18, 85-334-1047-6. 1.

Brener, B.; Lisboa, L.; Mattos, DPBG.; Arashiro, EKN.; Millar, PR.; Sudre, AP.; Duque, V. 2005. Frequência de enteroparasitas em amostras fecais de cães e gatos dos municípios do Rio de Janeiro e Niterói. *Revista Brasileira de Ciência Veterinária*. Vol. 12, Nº.1, janeiro-dezembro 2005, pp. 102-105, 1413-0130.

Bresciani, KDS.; Costa, AJ., Nunes, CM.; Serrano, ACM.; Moura, AB.; Stobbe, NS.; Perri, SHV.; Dias, RA.; Genari, SM. 2007. Ocorrência de anticorpos contra *Neospora caninum e Toxoplasma gondii* e estudo de fatores de risco em cães de Aracatuba – SP. *Ars Veterinária*. Vol. 23, Nº. 1, 2007, pp. 40-46, 0102-6380.

Bresciani, KDS.; Amarante, AFT.; Lima, VFM.; Feitosa, MM.; Feitosa, FLF.; Serrano, ACM.; Ishizaki, MN.; Tome, RO.; Táparo, CV.; Perri, SHV.; Meireles, MV. 2008. Infection by *Cryptosporidium* spp. in dogs from Araçatuba, SP, Brazil: Comparison between diagnostic methods and clinical and epidemiological analysis. *Veterinária e Zootecnia*. Vol. 15, Nº. 3, dezembro 2008, pp.466-468, 0102-5716.

Bresciani, KDS.; Costa, AJ.; Navarro, IT.; Toniolo, GH.; Sakamoto, CAM.; Arantes, TP.; Gennari, SM. 2008. Toxoplasmose canina: aspectos clínicos e patológicos. Semina: *Ciências Agrárias*, Londrina, Vol. 29, Nº. 1, jan./mar. 2008, pp. 189-202, 1679-0359.

Bresciani, KDS.; Costa, AJ.; Toniollo, GH.; Sabatini, GA.; Moraes, FR.; Paulillo, AC.; Ferraudo, AS. 1999. Experimental toxoplasmosis in pregnant bitches. *Veterinary Parasitology*, Amsterdam. Vol.86, Nº.2, 1999, pp.143-145, 0304-4017.

Bresciani, KDS.; Costa, AJG.; Toniollo, GH.; Luvizzoto, MCR.; Kanamura, CT.; Moraes, FR.; Perri, SHV.; Gennari, MS. 2009. Transplacental transmission of *Toxoplasma gondii* in reinfected pregnant female canines. *Parasitolology Research*. Vol. 1044, 2009, pp.1213–1217, 1432-1955.

Bresciani, KDS.; Toniollo, GH.; Costa, AJ.; Sabatini, GA.; Moraes, FR. 2001. Clinical, parasitological and obstetric observations in pregnant bitches with experimental toxoplasmosis. *Ciência Rural*, Santa Maria. Vol.31, Nº.6, 2001. pp.1039-1043, 0103-8478.

Brito, AF.; Souza, LC.; Silva, AV.; Langoni, H. 2002. Epidemiological and serological aspects in canine toxoplasmosis in animals with nervous symptoms. *Memórias do Instituto Oswaldo Cruz*, Rio de Janeiro. Vol.97, Nº.1, 2002, pp.31-35, 0074-0276.

Brooker, S.; Bethony, J.; Hotez, PJ. 2004. Human hookworm infection in the 21st Century. *Advances in Parasitology*. Vol. 58, 2004, pp. 197-288. 0065-308X.

Cañón-Franco, WA.; Bergamaschi, DP.; Labruna, MB.; Camargo, LM.; Silva, JC.; Pinter, A.; Gennari, SM. 2004. Ocurrence of anti-*Toxoplasma gondii* antibodies in dogs in the urban área of Monte Negro, Rondônia, Brazil. *Veterinary Research Communications*, Amsterdam, Vol.28, Nº.2, 2004, pp.113-118, 0165-7380.

Caumes,E. 2006. It's time to distinguish the sign "creeping eruption" from the syndrome"cutaneous larva migrans". *Dermatology*. Vol. 213, Nº. 3, 2006, pp. 179-81, 1018-8665.

Chieffi, PP.; Muller, EE. 1976. Prevalência de parasitismo por *Toxocara canis* em cães e presença de ovos de *Toxocara* sp no solo de localidades publicas da zona urbana do município de Londrina, estado do Paraná, Brasil. *Revista de Saúde Pública*. Vol. 10, Nº. 10, 1976, pp. 367-372. 0034-8910.

Coelho, NMD. 2009. *Ocorrência de cryptosporidium spp. em crianças e seus respectivos cães e gatos de estimação no Município de Andradina, SP*. Dissertação (Mestrado em Ciência Animal - Medicina Veterinária Preventiva e Produção Animal), Universidade Estadual Paulista. Araçatuba, SP.

Coelho, W. M. D.; Amarante, A. F. T.; Apolinario, J.C.; Coelho, N. M. D.; and Bresciani, K. D. S. Prevalence of Ancylostoma among dogs, cats and public places from Andradina city, São Paulo State,Brazil. *Revista do Instituto de Medicina Tropical de São Paulo* (in press), 2011. 0036- 4665.

Dubey, JP. 1985. Toxoplasmosis in dogs. *Canine Practice*. Vol.28, 1985, pp. 7-28, 0094-4904.

Dubey JP, Lindsay DS, Lappin MR. Toxoplasmosis and other intestinal coccidial infections in cats and dogs. *Veterinary Clinical Small Animal*. Vol. 39, 2009, pp. 1009-34.

Fayer R.; Trout, JM.; Xiao L.; Morgan, UM.; Lal, AA.; Dubey JP. 2001. *Cryptosporidium canis* from domestic dogs. *Journal Parasitology*. Vol. 87, 2001, pp. 1415-1422, 1937-2345.

Fayer R. 2010. Taxonomy and species delimitation in Cryptosporidium. *Experimental Parasitology*. Vol. 124, No. 1, january 2010, pp. 90-97, 0014-4894.

Frenkel, JK.; Parker, BB. 1996. An apparent role of dogs in the transmission of *Toxoplasma gondii* . The probable importance of xenosmophilia. *Annals of the New York Academy of Sciences*, New York. Vol.791, 1996, pp. 402-407, 1749-6632.

Fortes, E. 2004. *Parasitologia Veterinaria.* Editora: Ícone, 4ª Ed.; 9788527407779.

Gennari, SM.; Pena, HFJ.; Blasques, LS. 2001. Frequência de ocorrência de parasitos gastrintestinais em amostras de fezes de cães e gatos da cidade de São Paulo. *Veterinary News*, Vol. 8, Nº. 52, 2001, pp. 10-12.

Glickman, LT.; Schantz, PM. 1981. Epidemiology and pathogenesis of zoonotic toxocariasis. *Epidemiologic Reviews*, Vol. 3, 1981, pp. 230-250. 0193-936X.

Greene, CE. 1990. *Infectious diseases of the dog and cat.* Philadelphia: W. B. Saunders, 1990, pp.819-829, 9781-4160-3600-5.

Hammes, IS.; Gjerde, BJ.; Robertson, LJ. 2007. A longitudinal study on the occurrence of *Cryptosporidium* and *Giardia* in dogs during their first year of life. *Acta Veterinari Scandinavica.* Vol. 49, 2007, pp 1-10, 0044-605X.

Heukelbach, J.; Jackson, A.; Ariza, L.; et al. 2008. Prevalence and risk factors of hookworm-related cutaneous larva migrans in a rural community in Brazil. *Annals of Tropical Medicine and Parasitology*. Vol. 102, 2008, pp.53-61, 0003-4983.

Hoff, NP; Mota, R; Grofik, A; Hengge, UR. Cutaneous larva migrans. Vol. 59, 2008, pp 622-626, 0044-605X.

Jones, JL., Dietz, VJ., Power, M., et al. 2001. Survey of obstetrician-23. gynecologists in the United States about toxoplasmosis. *Infectious Diseases in Obstetrics and Gynecology*. Nº9, 2001, pp. 23-31, 1098-0097.

Prandota, J. 2010. Neuropathological changes and clinical features of autism spectrum disorder participants are similar to that reported in congenital and chronic cerebral toxoplasmosis in humans and mice. *Research in Autism Spectrum Disorders*, Vol. 4, Nº. 2, 2010, pp. 103-118, 1750-9467.

Lafferty, KD. 2005. Look what the cat dragged in: Do parasites contribute to human cultural diversity? *Behavioural Processes, Amsterdam*. Vol. 68, Nº.3, 2005, pp. 279-282, 0376-6357.

Laison, R.; Shaw, JJ.; Silveira, FT.; Braga, R. 1987. American visceral leishmaniasis: on the origin of Leishmania (Leishmania) chagasi. *Transactions of the Royal Society of Tropical Medicine and Hygiene*. Vol. 81, 1987, pp. 517, 0035-9203.

Lallo, MA.; Bondan, EF. 2006. Prevalência de *Criptosporidium* em cães de instituições da cidade de São Paulo. *Revista de Saúde Publica*. Vol. 40, 2006, pp. 120-125, 0034-8910.

Landmann, JK.; Prociv, P. 2003. Experimental human infection with the dog hookworm, *Ancylostoma caninum*. *Medical Journal of Australia*. Vol. 178, 2003, pp. 69-71. 0025-729X.

Lappin, MR. 2004. Doenças causadas por protozoários. In: ETTINGER, SJ.; FELDMAN, EC. (Ed.). *Tratado de medicina interna veterinária*: doenças do cão e do gato. 5.ed. Rio de Janeiro: Guanabara Koogan, 2004. pp. 430-435.

Lee, RJ. 1874. Case of creeping eruption. Transactions of the Clinical Society. Vol. 8, 1874, pp. 44-45, 0963-5157.

Lima, VMF.; Ikeda, FA.; Rossi, CN.; Feitosa, MM.; Vasconcelos, RO.; Nunes, CM.; Goto, H. 2010. Diminished CD4+/CD25+ T cell and increased IFN-γ levels occur in dogs vaccinated with Leishmune R in an endemic area for visceral leishmaniasis. *Veterinary Immunology and Immunopathology*. Vol. 135, 2010, pp. 296–302, 0165-2427.

Lima, VMF.; Biazzono, L.; Silva, AC.; Correa, APFL.; Luvizotto, MCR. 2005. Serological diagnosis of visceral leishmaniasis by an enzyme immunoassay using protein A in naturally infected dogs. *Pesquisa Veterinaria Brasileira*. Vol. 25, N°.4, 2005, pp. 215-218, 0100-736X.

Lindoso, JAL.; and Goto, H. 2006. Leishmaniose Visceral: situação atual e perspectivas futuras. *Boletim Epidemiológico Paulista*, Vol. 3, N° 26, 2006, 1806 -423-X.

Lindsay, DS.; Dubey, JP.; Butler, JM.; Blagburn, BL. 1997. Mechanical transmission of *Toxoplasma gondii* oocysts by dogs. *Veterinary Parasitology,* Amsterdam, Vol.73, N°.1/2, 1997, pp.27-33, 0304-4017.

Miller, NL.; Frenkel, JK.; Dubey, JP. 1972. Oral infections with Toxoplasma cysts and oocysts in felines, other mammals and birds. *Journal of Parasitology*, Vol.58, N°.5, 1972, pp.928-937, 1937-2345.

Monteiro, EM.; Silva, JCF.; Costa, RT.; Costa, DC.; Barata, RA.; Paula, EV.; Machado-Coelho, G. L. L.; Rocha, MF.; Fortes-Dias, C. L.; DIAS, E. D. 2005. Leishmaniose visceral: estudo de flebotomíneos e infecção canina em Montes Claros, Minas Gerais. *Revista da Sociedade Brasileira de Medicina Tropical*. Vol. 38, N°. 2, 2005, pp.147-152, 0037-8682.

Moro, FCB.; Pradebon, JB.; Santos, HT.; Querol, E. 2008. Ocorrência de *Ancylostoma* spp. e *Toxocara* spp. em praças e parques públicos dos municípios de Itaqui e Uruguaiana Fronteira oeste do Rio Grande do Sul. Biodiversidade Pampeana. Vol.6, 2008, pp.25-29, 1679-6179.

Mundim, MJS.; Rosa, LAG.; Hortencio, SM.; Faria, ESM.; Rodrigues, RM.; Curi, MC. 2007. Prevalence of *Giardia duodenalis* and *Cryptosporidium* spp. in dogs from different living conditions in Uberlandia, Brazil. *Veterinary Parasitology.* Vol. 144, 2007, pp. 356-359, 0304-4017.

Netto, LC.; Lima, F F.; Perri, SHV.; Koivisto, M.; Bresciani. 2011. Programa de conscientização de idosos sobre posse responsável de animais de estimação em bairro periférico do município de Araçatuba, SP. *Revista Ciência em Extensão* Vol. 7, 2011, pp. 102-109, 1679-4605.

Ogassawara, S.; Benassi, S.; Larsson, CE.; Leme, PTZ.; Hagiwara, MK. 1986. Prevalência de infecções helmínticas em gatos na cidade de São Paulo. *Revista da Faculdade de Medicina Veterinária e Zootecnia da Universidade de São Paulo.* Vol.23, 1986, pp.145-149, 0303-7525.

Oppermann, WH. Versuche zum experimentellen infection des hundes mit Toxoplasma - oozysten. 1971. Dissertation (Mestrado) - Institute fur Parasitologie des Fachbereiches Veterinarmedizin, Universität Berlin, Berlin.

Overgaauw, PAM. 1997. Aspects of *Toxocara* epidemiology: human toxocarosis. *Critical Reviews in Microbiology.* Vol. 23, N°. 3, 1997, pp. 215-231, 1473-5601.

Paranhos, S M.; Freitas, L.; Santos, WC.; Grimaldi Jr, G.; Pontes, C LC.; Oliveira, SAA. 1996. Cross-sectional serodiagnostic survey of canine leishmaniasis due to *Leishmania chagasi. American Journal of Tropical Medicine and Hygiene.* Vol. 55, 1996, pp. 39-44, 0002-9637.

Pfukenyi, DM.; Chipunga, SL.; Dinginya, L.; Matenga, E. 2010. A survey of pet ownership,wareness, and public knowledge of pet zoonoses with particular reference to roundworms and hookworms in Harare, Zimbabwe. *Tropical Animal Health and Production.* Vol. 42, 2010, pp. 247-252, 1573-7438.

Plutzer J, and Karanis, P. 2009. Genetic polymorphism in Cryptosporidium species: in update. *Veterinary Parasitology.* Vol. 165, No. 3-4, pp. 187-199, 0304-4017.

Pradhan, S.; Yadav, R.; Mishra, VN. 2007. Toxoplasma meningoencephalitis in HIV-seronegative patients: clinical patterns, imaging features and treatment outcome. *Transactions of the Royal Society of Tropical Medicine and Hygiene*, London. Vol.101, N°.1, pp.25-33, 0035- 9203.

Rossignol, JF. 2010. *Cryptosporidium* and *Giardia*: treatment options and prospects for new drugs. *Experimental Parasitology.* Vol. 124, 2010, pp. 45-53, 0014-4894.

Rosypal, AC.; Corte's-Vecino, JA.; Genarri, SM.; Dubey, JP.; Tidwell, RR.; Lindsay, DS. 2007. Serological survey of *Leishmania infantum* and *Trypanosoma cruzi* in dogs from urban areas of Brazil and Colombia. *Veterinary Parasitoogy.* Vol. 149, 2007, pp. 172-177, 0103-846X.

Santarém, VA.; Giuffrida, R.; and Zanin, AZ. 2004. Larva migrans cutânea: ocorrência de casos humanos e identificação de larvas de Ancylostoma spp. em parque público do município de Taciba, São Paulo. *Revista da Sociedade Brasileira de Medicina Tropical.* Vol. 37, Nº. 2, march-april 2004, pp. 179-181, 0037-8682.

Santos, TR.; Nunes, CM.; Luvizotto, MCR.; Moura, AB.; Lopes, WDZ.; Costa, AJ.; Bresciani, KDS. Detection of Toxoplasma gondii oocysts in environmental samples from public schools. *Veterinary Parasitology.* Vol.171, Nº.1, 2010, pp.53–57,0103-846X.

São Paulo (ESTADO). Secretaria de Estado da Saúde. Superintendência de Controle de Endemias – SUCEN e Coordenadoria de Controle de Doenças–CCD. *Manual de Vigilância e Controle da Leishmaniose Visceral Americana do Estado de São Paulo.* São Paulo, 2006. pp.158.

Schares, G.; Pantchev, N.; Barutzki, D.; Heydorn, AO.; Bauer, C; Conraths, FJ. 2005. Oocysts of *Neospora caninum*, *Hammondia heydorni*, *Toxoplasma gond*ii and *Hammondia hammondi* in faeces collected from dogs in Germany. *International Jounal for Parasitology*, Oxford. Vol. 35, Nº.14, 2005, pp.1525-1537, 0020-7519.

Silva, ES.; Gontijo, CM.; Pirmez, C.; Fernandes, O.; Brazil, RP. 2001. Short report: detection of *Leishmania* DNA by polymerase chain reaction on blood samples from dogs with visceral leishmaniasis. *American Journal of Tropical Medicine and Hygiene.* Vol. 65, Nº.6, 2001, pp. 896-898, 0002-9637.

Smith, RP., Chalmers, KE., Elwin, K., Clifton-Hadley, A., Mueller-Doblies, D., Watkins, J., Paiba, GA., Giles, M. 2009. Investigation the role of companion animals in the zoonotic transmission of cryptosporidiosis. *Zoonoses and Public Health.* Vol. 56, No. 1, february 2009, pp. 24-33, 1863-1959.

Soares, JAS.; Nasser, LS.; Carvalho, SFG.; Caldeira, AP. 2011. Achados oculares em crianças com toxoplasmose congênita. *Aruivos Brasileiros de Oftalmologia.* [online]. Vol.74, Nº.4, pp. 255-257. ISSN 0004-2749.

Souza, SLP.; Gennari, SM.; Yai, LEO.; D'auria, SRN.; Cardoso, SMS.; Guimarães JJS.; Dubey, JP. 2003. Ocurrence of *Toxoplasma gondii* antibodies in sera from dogs of the urban and rural areas from Brazil.

Revista Brasileira de Parasitologia Veterinária, São Paulo. Vol.12, Nº.1, 2003, pp.1-3, 1984-2961.

Táparo, CV.; Perri, SHV.; Serrano, ACM.; Ishizaki, MN.; Costa, TP.; Amarante, AFT.; Bresciani, KDS. 2006. Comparação entre técnicas coproparasitológicas no diagnóstico de ovos de helmintos e oocistos de protozoários em cães. *Revista Brasileira de Parasitologia Veterinária*. Vol. 15, No. 1, 2006, pp. 1-5, 1984-2961.

Thomaz, A.; Meireles, MV.; Soares, RM.; Pena, HFJ.; Gennari, SM. 2007. Molecular identification of *Cryptosporidium* spp. from fecal samples of felines, canines and bovines in the state of Sao Paulo, Brazil. *Veterinary Parasitology*. Vol. 150, 2007, pp. 291-296, 0304-4017.

Thompson, RCA., Palmer, CS., and O´Handley, R. 2008. The public health and clinical significance of Giardia and Cryptosporidium in domestic animals. *The Veterinary Journal*. Vol. 177, No. 1., july 2008, pp. 18-25, 1090-0233.

Tome, RO.; Serrano, ACM.; Nunes, CM.; Perri, SHV.; Bresciani, KDS. 2005. Inquerito epidemiológico sobre conceitos de zoonoses parasitárias para professores de escolas municipais do ensino infantil de Aracatuba-SP. *Revista Científica em Extensão*, Vol. 2, No.1, 2005, pp.38-46.

Troncarelli, MZ.; Machado, JG.; Camargo, LB.; Hoffmann, JL.; Camossi, L.; Greca, H.; Faccioli, PY.; Langoni, H. 2008. Associação entre resultados sorológicos no diagnóstico da leishmaniose e da tripanossomíase canina, pela técnica de imunofluorescência indireta. *Veterinaria e Zootecnia*. Vol. 15, Nº.1, 2008, pp. 40-47, 0102 -5716.

Tzipori, S.; and Griffths. 1998. Natural History and Biology of *Cryptosporidium parvum*. *Advances in Parasitology*. Vol. 40, 1998, pp. 4-36, 0065-308X.

Urquhart, GM.; Armour, J.; Duncan, JL.; Dunn, AM.; Jennings, FW. 1991. *Parasitologia Veterinária*. Rio de Janeiro : Guanabara Koogan, 1991. pp. 306, 1984-2961.

Vasconcellos, MC.; Barros, JSR.; Oliveira, CS. 2006. Parasitas gastrointestinais em cães institucionalizados no Rio de Janeiro, RJ. *Revista de Saúde Publica*, Vol. 40, pp. 321-323. 0034-8910.

Xiao, L.; Morgan, UM.; Josef, L.; Escalante, A.; Michael, A.; William, S.; Thompson, RCA.; Ronald, F.; Lal. AA. 1999. Genetic Diversity within *Cryptosporidium parvum* and related *Cryptosporidium* Species. *Appied and Microbiology Environmental*. Vol. 65, 1999, pp.3386-3391, 0099-2240.

Yacob, HT.; Ayele, T.; Fikru, R.; Basu, AK.; 2007. Gastrointestinal nematodes in dogs from Debre Zeit, Ethiopia. *Veterinary Parasitology*. Vol. 148: pp.144-148, 0103-846X.

In: Canine Behavior, Classification and Diseases ISBN: 978-1-62081-304-1
Editors: R. L. Andrade and C. I. Batista

Chapter V

Dog Bites: A Study of Victims, Injuries and Circumstances in the Southeast of Mexico

Matilde Jimenez-Coello[1], Karla Y. Acosta-Viana[1], Antonio Ortega Pacheco[3,], Eugenia Guzman-Marin[1], Luz M. Yanez-Gamboa[2] and Dario M. Guiris-Andrade[2]*

[1]CA. Biomedicina de Enfermedades Infecciosas y Parasitarias Laboratorio de Biología Celular, CIR 'Dr Hideyo Noguchi', Universidad Autónoma de Yucatán, Mérida, Yucatán, México

[2]Departamento de Medicina, Facultad de Medicina Veterinaria y Zootecnia, Universidad Autónoma de Chiapas, Tuxtla-E, Zapata, México

[3]Departamento de Salud Animal y Medicina Preventiva, Facultad de Medicina Veterinaria y Zootecnia, Universidad Autónoma de Yucatán, Mérida-Xmatkuil, Mérida, Yucatán, México

[*] Corresponding author: Tel.: +52 (999)924 57 55 ext. 120. Fax +52 (999)924 57 55. Email address: opacheco@uady.mx (A. Ortega-Pacheco).

Abstract

Dog bites in humans are a public health problem of worldwide distribution. As a result of human population growth, the absence of responsible dog ownership polices and the increased numbers of free-roaming dogs especially in developing countries, dog bite injuries in people are frequently reported.

The aim of this study was to determine the common regions of bites and to identify factors associated with dog bites in humans, in the city of Tuxtla Gutierrez, Chiapas, Mexico. A hospital-based questionnaire survey was conducted during 2007 among dog bites victims who visited a referral hospital (SSA) in the city of Tuxtla Gutierrez, Chiapas. A total of 194 persons were recorded. From those, 175 (89.7%) receive hospital care due to injuries caused by dog bites and 19 (10.3%) were attended by the bite of another domestic animal or wildlife species. Throughout the year, it was observed that the months with more cases of bites were mor frequently recorded during March and June matching with the official holiday periods in schools in Mexico.

The age of persons attacked in a higher proportion (61.7%) were in the age groups of 1-10, 11-20 and 21-30 years old. There was no difference in the gender of the victims attacked by dogs (50.9 and 49.1% for male and female gender respectively). The dog bite victims occurred more commonly in people with low educational level (elementary and junior high school) in comparison with higher educational levels. Places where people were attacked by dogs were in the households and the streets, in most cases by stray dogs. In relation to the number of injuries caused by dog attacks, 80.9% of cases were reported as multiple lesions (type II) and only 19% had a single lesion associated with the attack (type I).

The anatomic regions where victims were assaulted were in the legs, hands, feet and arms. From the dogs bitting people, 80.57% had owner and 19.4% were ownerless stray dogs. In addition to physical injuries, bites can potentially transmit a large number of zoonotic diseases (including rabies) to their victims. Increased educational awareness of people about the risk of dog bites is necessary together with enforcement of regulations for licensing of dogs, efficient stray dog population management and animal birth control programs to reduce bite incidents, especially in developing countries such as Mexico.

Keywords: Dog bite, injures, children, free roaming dogs

Introduction

Dog bites are a public health problem because of a large number of clinical complications in individuals attacked. It is especially important because of the potential transmission of multiple zoonotic infectious agents.

Each year, several million of Americans are bitten by animals, causing approximately 300,000 visits to emergency departments, 10,000 hospitalizations and 20 deaths, mostly among young children. Ninety percent of these bites are from dogs and cats, and bites become infected in 3-18% of the cases when caused by dogs and 28-80% when associated by cat bites. Occasional sequelaes of meningitis, endocarditis, septic arthritis, and septic shock are seen in those cases (Talan et al., 1999).

The growth of the canine population in Mexico is a serious problem as in many developing countries. Dogs are common pets in Southern Mexico as in many other regions of the country with a high density of dogs in both rural and urban areas (Ortega-Pacheco, 2001; Ortega-Pacheco et al., 2007). Dog bites are commonly reported in the country. In 2007 a total of 116.832 cases of dog bites were reported in the states of Durango, Hidalgo, Puebla, Mexico City and San Luis Potosi, where the most commonly affected victims were children under 15 years of age (Sistema Nacional de Vigilancia Epidemiológica, 2008).

The habits of dog owners, lack of respect for the laws governing the possession of dogs as well as the overpopulation of stray dogs are factors that act together to increase the problem of dog bites in Mexico. In Tuxtla Gutierrez, Chiapas, in a preliminary study a ratio dog: owner of 1:4 was found, demonstrating the high abundance of these species and close contact to people in the city (Güiris et al., 2007). This is an important risk factor that may predispose the aggression and biting of dogs in the inhabitants of the city.

The purpose of this chapter was to describe the epidemiological aspects of dog bites to people in an urban area of southeast Mexico to establish the knowledge that allows taking appropriate measures for the prevention and control in the population at risk. No previous reports of dog aggression are found in the state of Chiapas, Mexico.

Materials and Methods

Type of study: This cohort study includes the characteristics of dog bites and the characteristics presented by patients attacked in the city of Tuxtla

Gutierrez, Chiapas during the study period of one year (January to December 2007) that were attended at the municipal hospital of health services.

Study area: This study was performed in Tuxtla Gutierrez, capital city of the State of Chiapas, Mexico (93°07' and 16°45'N latitude, and 93°07´and 94°15´W longitude). The climate in the area is sub-humid with a well defined rainy season during the summer.

Studied population: The research focused on the individuals involved in the events of bites attended at the municipal center for health services (Secretaria de Salubridad y Asistencia SSA) for proper management and treatment of animal bites.

Statistical analysis: The results were analyzed using descriptive statistics to obtain the frequency identified from patients with a history of aggression. The proportions of being bitten was estimated according to age, gender, education, place of occurrence, anatomical lesion affected and type of injury Type I (single) or type II (multiple).

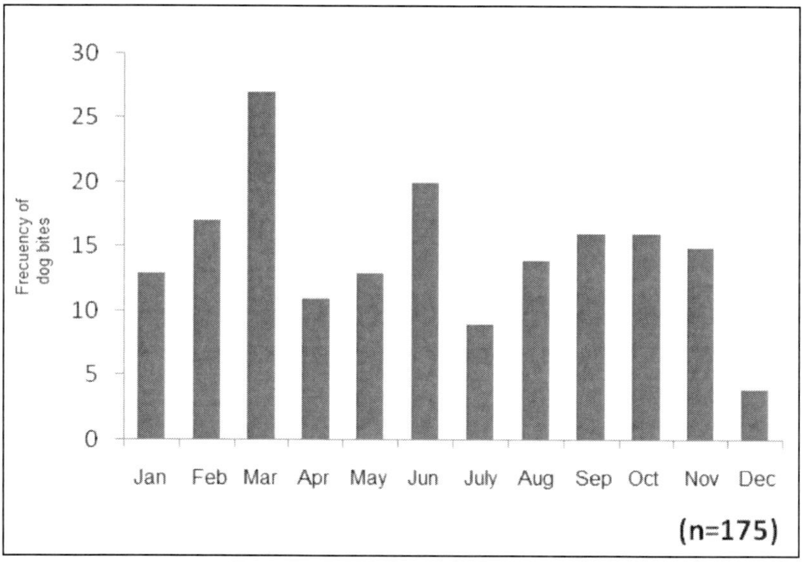

Figure 1. Annual distribution of dog bites reported from the Health Center of Tuxtla Gutierrez, Chiapas, during 2007.

Age of victims: Victims more commonly affected were those between 1 to 30 years old (108 cases, 61.7%). Only 67 cases (38.3%) were identified on people >31 years old (Figure 2). In relation to the gender of the victims, there were identified 89 cases of male and 86 female cases and corresponded to 50.9 and 49.1% respectively.

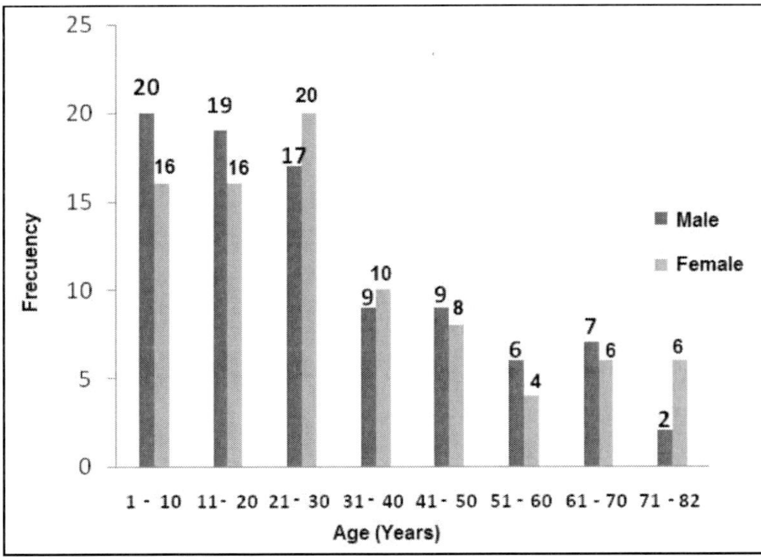

Figure 2. Frequency of dog bite cases in different age groups and gender.

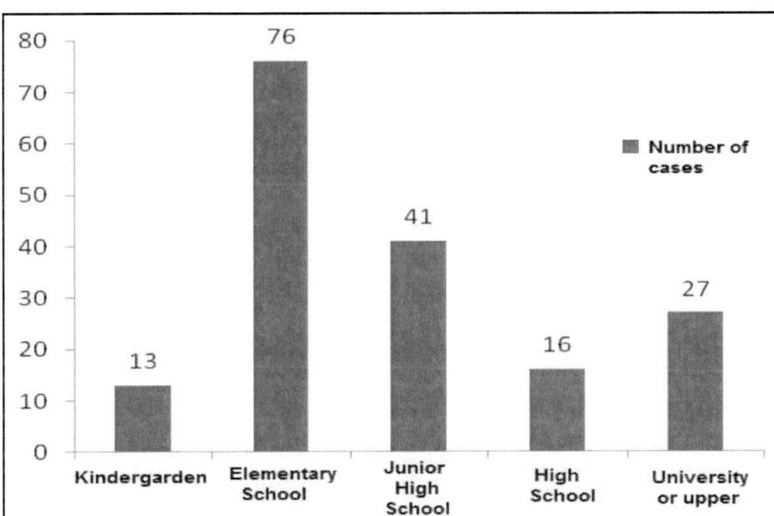

Figure 3. Educational level of the patients reported with dog bite injuries during 2007 in Tuxtla Gutierrez, Chiapas Mexico.

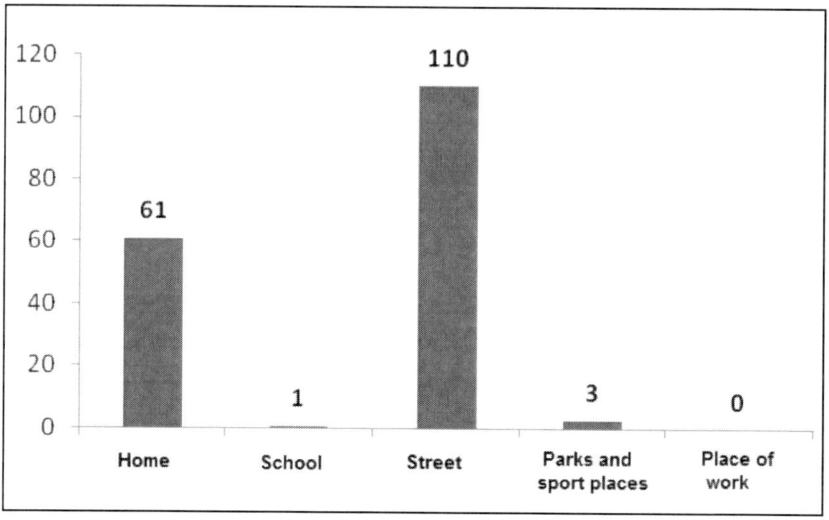

Figure 4. Place of occurrence where dog bites reported in patients who went to the hospital.

Education: According to the educational level of the victims, the individuals in the primary (elementary) school level (n=76) were the ones with a higher frequency of dog bites (44%) when compared to other groups (Figure 3).

Results

Frequency and monthly distribution of bites: From a total of 194 people bitten by an animal, 175 were associated with dog bite injuries (89.7%) and 19 (10.3%) were assaulted by other domestic and wild species. Throughout the year, a higher number of cases were observed during the months of March and June (Figure 1).

Place of occurrence: The places more frequently reported where the attacks occurs were on the streets (62.8% 110 cases) and at home (34.8% 61 cases) (Figure 4). Other reported places were at school, sports and sport places; none of the cases occurred at the place of work.

Type of injury and anatomic region affected. As for the type of injury produced by the dog bite, the vast majority (80.9%) of bites caused an injury classified as Type I (single) and only 19% of the assaults resulted in injuries classified as Type II (multiple) (Figure 5).

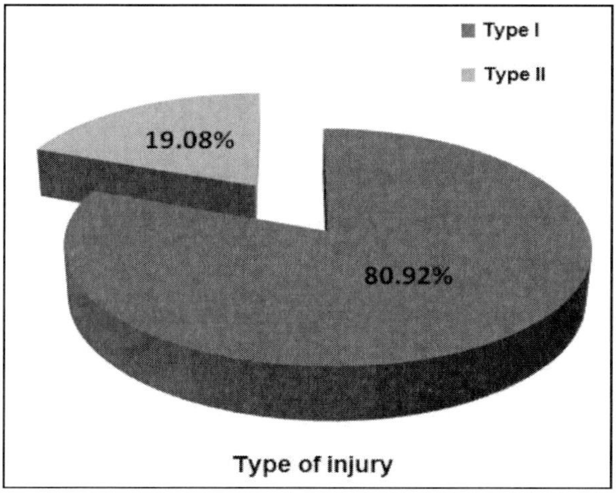

Figure 5. Types of injury caused by dog bite attack.

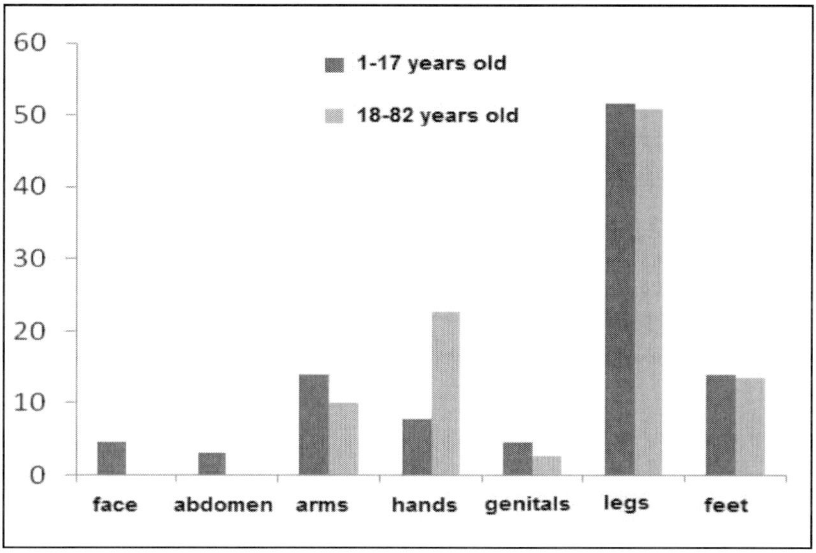

Figure 6. Anatomical regions affected by age groups who went to hospital care for dog bites in 2007.

The anatomical region most frequently affected in 49.1% (85 cases) were the legs; according to age group, children (1 to 17 years old) presented in addition to the leg injury, aggression on the face and abdomen 4.7% 3.1% respectively. Adults (18 to 80 years old) do not show lesion on these anatomical regions. Also, arms and genital bites were reported more frequently in children than in older individuals (Figure 6).

Table 1. Type of ownership of dogs that attacked people in Tuxtla Gutierrez Chiapas, during 2007

Type of dog		Frecuency	(%)
Identified	*Intra-domiciliary dog*	63	36.0
	Extra-domiciliary dog	78	44.6
Not identified		34	19.4
Total		175	100

As for the dogs that bite people 141 (80.6%) were identified owned dogs and 34 (19.4%) were recorded as unidentified. Identifiable dogs were those that have an owner, with free acces to the streets most of the day (free roaming owned dogs) (44.6%) and dogs kept indoors (36%) (intra-domiciliary owned dogs) (Table 1).

Discusion

Dog bites are an important and prevalent problem in the city of Tuxtla Gutierrez as in many other parts of Mexico and in the world. Similar works describe that dog bites are the most common cause of assaults by animals, corresponding to 90% of them (Gregory et al., 2005; Jofré et al., 2006; Eslamifar et al., 2008; Ichhpujani et al., 2008). Frequency of dog bites may increase every year if no preventive control measures are taken (Palacio et al., 2005; Sistema Nacional de Vigilancia Epidemiologica, 2008) especially focoused on the education of pet owners (Duprerrex et al., 2009). The veterinary consult is a perfect time to raise awareness among owners who often are not well informed about the behavior of their pets and have only limited knowledge on dogs; education should include body language and social cues to prevent dog bites especially in infants and toddlers (Reisner and Shofer, 2008).

Among the characteristics of attacker dogs identified during this study no differences were observed by gender indicating that the risk of aggression is the same regardless of sex. Similar findings have benn reported by Gregory et al., (2005) but contrary to that described by O'Sullivan et al., (2008) who found that in Ireland male dogs have a higher proportion of owner-bite attacks. These differences may be due to several issues from each country or even within a country regarding the structure of dog population, cultural relationships between dogs and owners and many other risk factors; for instance a female dog raisng puppies may be very aggressive during this time towards people approaching them. In this study, younger persons (<30 years) were observed with greater risk of being bite similarly as described in multiple studies of dog bites from different parts of the world (Thomas and Buntine, 1987; Gandhi et al., 1999; Lavaud et al., 2005; Hemmo-Lotem et al., 2006; Reisner and Shofer 2008; Ichhpujani et al., 2008; Zanini et al., 2008; Rosado et al., 2008; Monroy et al., 2009).

Other identified risk factos found in this study included the months of the year, age and education level of bite victims. The month of the year when bites were more frequently reported happen together with the official holiday periods in Mexico; probably because children stay longer periods of time with their dogs increasing the risk of assault. Similar pattern of dog bites during holiday periods is also found in Spain (Rosado et al., 2009) and USA (Monroy et al., 2009).

Although most of dog offenders were owned, were also identified as extradomiciliary because they were were free roaming most of the day. A similar situation is also described by Thompson (1997); Tuncali et al., (2005), Schwartzman and Pacin (2005) and Zanini et al., (2008). The house was the second important places where dog bites occurred. Schavartzman and Pacin (2005) found that more than half of dog bites (62%) occur within the limits of the house belonging to dog owners as in the present study.

The age of the children bitten whitin the house was lower than children bitten in the street. Youngest children spend more time at home and in the wish for playing with their pet (dogs in this case) they may react negatively so a greatest risk of bites is expected; thus appropriate measures may be primarily focoused towards this age group. By contrast with children from elementary and Junior High school for their activities, they stay more time away from home and are having lower probability of been biten by their own dogs. However, are at risk of being bitten on public highways. Other sites where dog bites may occur is in schools, recreational and sports centers, etc. but were uncommon in this study. In Trinidad and Tobago where free roaming dogs are abundant dog bites in childrens are common events recorded outside their homes (Georges and Adesiyun, 2008). A practical guide according to every region situation should be implemented and be available for families with young children to prevent exposure to free roaming dogs and prevent bites. These require the identification of potentially dangerous dog near children homes (Avner and Baker, 1991).

In the present study dog bite injuries were mostly in the legs from both adults and children over 10 years old. Only children <5 years were attend for face and abdomen injuries. These findings slightly differ to those described by Gandhi et al., (1999) who found that dog bite injuries in children occurs more frequently in the head and neck followed by injuries in the limbs and less frequently in other parts of the body. The results of this investigation correspond to those described by Hemmo-Lotem et al., (2006) who states that in Israel the extremities are more often affected (64%) and the region of the head and neck is assaulted in a smaller proportion (27%). In Latin America, Zanini et al., (2008) also agrees with the findings of this study. They reported a higher dog bite proportion of the lower extremities (55%) compared to those recorded in the head-neck region (11%). The correspondence in these findings could be due to a similarity in the Latin American culture of dog ownership and dog-person relationship unlike in the Middle East or elsewhere. The neighborhood in the city of Tuxtla Gutierrez where more cases of people bitten by dogs occurred was located in the north east region, probably this is because it is a poor urban area with a high proportion of families with a low average income economic index and is associated with a high percentage of stray dogs and owned dogs wandering in the street. Families in other cities from southern Mexico with a middle-low economic income have a significantly higher number of dogs which likely leads to increased dog population in that area and therefore a greater risk of aggression (Ortega-Pacheco et al., 2007). Abundance of dogs in the streets is higly associated with bites to humans. In Okayama, Japan, the density of 225 stray dogs/km^2 and a proportion of dog to humans of 1:5.2 found in that area was considered an important risk of dog bites (Kato et al., 2003).

It is important to mention that in many cases of dog bites people do not take medical supervision because they do not give importance to such incidents and/or ignore the risk of contracting a disease transmitted by dog bites. Probably this is because 80% of bite injuries are type I, because of this, patients underestimate the potential health risks. A proper medical treatment should include an appropriate wound care and under the conditions of developing countries the consideration of free vaccination against rabies. Preventing dog bites requires measures aimed at dog owners, parents, children and local authorities.

Conclusion

Dog bites is a common and important public health problem in the city of Tuxtla Gutierrez Chiapas, Mexico. Dog bite victims have the potential risk of developing infection diseases by multiple microorganisms transmitted in the saliva of dogs including rabies. Associated factors described in this study should be taken into account to prevent bites in the studied area. It is necessary to establish adequate control measures to prevent or decrease the number of dog bites in joint collaboration between government authorities, veterinarians and pet owners especially among young people.

References

Avner JR, Baker MD, (1991) Dog bites in urban children. *Pediatrics*, 88:55-57.

Duperrex O., Blackhall K, Burri M, Jeannot E., (2009). Education of children and adolescents for the prevention of dog bite injuries. *Cochrane Database Syst. Rev*. 15:CD004726. Review.

Eslamifar Ali, Ramezani Amitis, Razzaghi-Abyaneh Mehdi, Fallahian Vida, Mashayekhi Parisa, Hazrati Mahbood, Azkari Tina, Fayaz Ahmad, Aghakhani Arezoo. (2008) Animal Bites in Tehran, Iran. *Arch. Iran Med.* 11:200-202.

Gandhi RR, Liebman MA, Staffort BL, Staford PW. (1999) Dog bites injuries in children: a preliminary survey. *Am. Surg*. 65:863-864.

Georges K., Adesiyun A. (2008) An investigation into the prevalence of dog bites to primary school children in Trinidad. *BCM Public Health*, 8: 1-7.

Gregory PA., Eeckhout V., Wylock P. (2005) Dog bites: an overview, *Eur. J. Plasr. Surg.*, 28:233-238.

Güiris ADM., Martínez FL., Yáñez GLM., Pérez E.M.E., Oliva LL. (2007) Riesgo Parasítico por Fauna en la ciudad de Tuxtla Gutiérrez, Chiapas. Unidad de Vinculación Docente, Fac. de MVZ., UNACH, pp. 1-16.

Hemmo-Lotem M., Barnea Y., Jinich-Aronowits C., Endy-Findling L., Leshem D., Zaratski A., Merrick J. (2006) Epidemiology of pediatric bite/sting injuries. One-year study of pediatric emergency department in Israel. *Scientific World Journal*. 6:653-660.

Ichhpujani RL., Mala C., Veena M., Singh J., Bhardwaj M., Bhattacharya D., Pattanaik SK., Balakrishnan N., Reddy AK., Samnpath G., Gandhi N.,

Nagar SS., Shiy L. (2008) Epidemiology of animal bites and rabies cases in India. A multicentric study. *J. Commun. Dis.* 40: 27-36.

Jofré ML., Perret PC., Abarca KV., Solari VG., Olivares CR., López Del PJ. (2006) Recomendaciones para el manejo de mordeduras ocasionadas por animales. *Rev. Chil. Infect.* 23:20-34.

Kato M., Hideki Y., Yoshihide I., Shohei K. (2003) Survey of the stray dog population and the Health Education Program on the prevention of dog bites and dog-acquired infections: A comparative study in Nepal and Okayama prefecture, Japan. *Acta Med. Okayama.* 57:261-266.

Lavaud J., Vazquez MP., Bordas VC., Duval C. (2005) Domestic animals and accidents in children. *Arch. Pediatr.* 12:228-233.

Monroy A., Behar P., Nagy M., Poje C., Pizzuto M., Brodsky L. (2009) Head and neck dog bites in children. *Otolaryngol. Head Neck Surg.* 140:354-357.

Ortega-Pacheco A., Rodriguez-Buenfil JC., Bolio-Gonzalez M., Sauri-Arceo CH., Jiménez-Coello M., Forsberg CL. (2007) A Survey of Dog Populations in Urban and Rural Areas of Yucatan, Mexico. *Anthrozoos.* 20:261-274.

Ortega-Pacheco A. (2001) La sobrepoblación canina: un problema con repercusiones potenciales para la salud humana. *Rev. Biomed.* 12:290-291.

O'Sullivan EN., Jones BR., O'Sullivan K., Hanlon AJ. (2008) Characteristics of 234 dog bite incidents in Ireland during 2004 and 2005. *Vet. Rec.* 163:34-42.

Palacio J., León M., García S. (2005) Aspectos epidemiológicos de las mordeduras de perro. España. *Gac. Sanit.* 19:50-58.

Reisner IR., Shofer FS. (2008) Effects of gender and parental status on knowledge and attitudes of dog owners regarding dog aggression toward children. *J. Am. Vet. Med. Assoc.* 233:1412-1419.

Rosado B., García-Belenguer S., León M., Palacio J. (2009) A comprehensive study of dog bites in Spain, 1995-2004. *Vet. J.* 179:383-391.

Schvartzman DS., Pacín BM. (2005) Lesiones por mordeduras de perros en niños. *Arch. Argent. Pediatr.* 103:389-395.

Sistema Nacional de Vigilancia Epidemiológica (2008) Secretaría de Salud Mordedura por perro problema de salud pública (segunda y última parte), *Epidemiología*, 25:1-4. Available at http://www.dgepi.salud. gob. mx/boletin/2008/sem38/pdf/edit3808.pdf.

Talan DA., Citron DM., Abrahamian FM., Moran GJ., Goldstein EJC. (1999) Bacteriologic analysis of infected dog and cat bites. *New England J. Med.* 340:85-92.

Thomas PR., Buntine JA. (1987) Man's best friend?: A review of the Austin Hospital's experience with dog bites. *Med. J. Aust.* 147:536-540.

Thompson GP. (1997) The public health impact of dog attacks in a major Australian city. *Med. J. Australia.* 6:29-32.

Tuncali D., Bingul F., Terzioglu A., Aslan G., (2005) Animal bites. *Saudi Med. J.* 26:772-776.

Zanini F., Padinger P., Elisondo Ma. C., Pérez H. (2008) Epidemiología de las lesiones por mordedura de perro en Tierra del Fuego, Argentina. *Medicina (Buenos Aires).* 68: 1-5.

In: Canine Behavior, Classification and Diseases ISBN: 978-1-62081-304-1
Editors: R. L. Andrade and C. I. Batista

Chapter VI

Genetics of Dog Behavior*

***Linda van den Berg*[1,2], *Diane van Rooy*[3] *and Claire Wade*[3]**
[1]Department of Pediatrics and [2]Human Genetics, Leiden University Medical Center, Leiden, The Netherlands
[3]Faculty of Veterinary Science, The University of Sydney, Australia

Abstract

All modern dog breeds are descendants of the grey wolf. Dogs were originally selected for behavioral traits: dogs have been bred to guard, herd, hunt, pull sledges, and to provide companionship. Early canid domestication involved selection for tameness. Studies of silver foxes at the Institute of Cytology and Genetics in Novosibirsk have shown that a few generations of selection for tameness can lead to a domesticated strain of foxes that not only show dog-like behaviors, but that also display phenotypic traits such as curly tails, drop ears, and loss of pigment. The early domestication of dogs was followed by the formation of dog breeds much later. Extreme founder effects, drift, and selection for novelty, in combination with genetic isolation during breed formation, have resulted

* A version of this chapter also appears in Dogs: Biology Behavior and Health Disorders, edited by Vincent M. DeGiovine, published by Nova Science Publishers, Inc. It was submitted for appropriate modifications in an effort to encourage wider dissemination of research.

in a canine genome sequence with features that are highly favorable for the molecular genetic study of inherited traits. Long linkage disequilibrium within breeds and a limited number of short common haplotypes across breeds greatly facilitate gene mapping. Canine genomic tools such as microarrays for genotyping and gene expression studies have enabled the identification of causal mutations for several canine morphological and disease susceptibility traits in recent years. In this review chapter, we discuss the latest knowledge regarding the inheritance of behavioral traits in dogs. We also describe molecular genetic studies that have pinpointed some genetic variants that contribute to behavior. Behavioral traits that are discussed are canine personality, working behavior, anxiety, aggression, obsessive-compulsive disorder, and feeding behavior.

1. Introduction

Domestic dogs display a fascinating morphological variation that is unique among mammals. For instance, the difference in size between chihuahuas and great danes is almost a 100-fold. Quantitative trait loci (QTLs, i.e. stretches of DNA that contain genes that affect a quantitative trait) for several breed-defining traits have been identified in the past few years, including skeletal traits (Parker *et al.* 2009; Sutter *et al.* 2007), hair characteristics (Cadieu *et al.* 2009; Drögemüller *et al.* 2008; Salmon Hillbertz *et al.* 2007), coat color (Candille *et al.* 2007; Karlsson *et al.* 2007), and wrinkled skin (Akey *et al.* 2010).

For several of these traits, the causal genetic variant has been identified (e.g. a premature stop codon in the melanocyte-stimulating hormone receptor gene in Labrador and golden retrievers with yellow coat color, Everts *et al.* 2000).

Dog breeds also differ in behavioral characteristics. An example is the different attitude of guarding breeds and herding breeds towards livestock as described by Spady and Ostrander (2008). Herding breeds like border collies have been selected to manage the movement and behavior of livestock. These dogs express predatory behavior such as circling, crouching and eye. Guarding breeds like the maremma have been selected to live among livestock and to guard against predators. They usually do not show predatory behaviors. Scott and Fuller (1965) performed an influential study of breed differences and hereditary aspects of canine behavior.

Their experiment involved 470 dogs of five breeds: basenji, beagle, American cocker spaniel, Shetland sheepdog and wire haired fox terrier. Breeds and their crosses were compared for reactivity, trainability and problem-solving behaviors. Scott and Fuller observed behavioral differences between the breeds in the majority of their behavioral tests. For instance, there were breed differences in playful aggression and dominance.

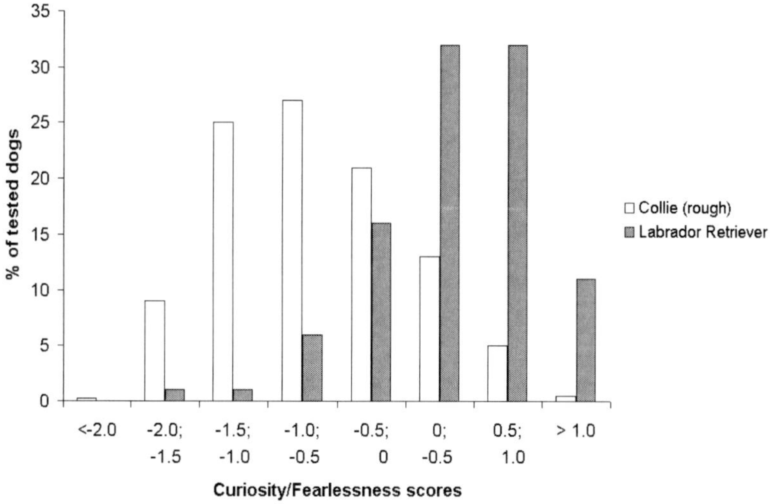

Figure 1. This figure shows a result of the study of breed-typical behaviour by Svartberg (2006). The distribution of curiosity/fearlessness scores is shown for two dog breeds: collies and Labrador retrievers. Labradors were the highest ranking breed for this trait and collies ranked the lowest. It is clearly visible that, although there is a lot of variation within the breeds, the means of the distributions of the breeds are shifted with respect to each other. (Figure reprinted from Svartberg 2006 with permission from Elsevier).

Wire haired fox terriers were the most aggressive. The terrier puppies consistently "ganged up" on group members. These attacks were so serious that victims had to be removed in order to prevent serious injury. More recently, Svartberg (2006) compared the behavior of 31 breeds using data from a standard behavioral test from 13097 dogs. The study observed significant differences between the breeds in all investigated traits. However, both Scott and Fuller (1965) and Svartberg (2006) reported large variation within the breeds (Figure 1).

It is believed that dogs were originally selected for behavioral traits. Dogs have been selected to guard, herd, hunt, pull sledges, and to provide companionship. Later, particularly in the Victorian era, selection for appearance became more important. The fact that breed differences in behavior are observed and that these observed behavioral dispositions can be selected for, suggests that there is a genetic basis for the individual variation in behavior. So far, the identification of genetic variants that affect canine behavior has lagged behind the identification of genetic variants for morphological traits and somatic diseases. In this chapter, we will review the latest knowledge concerning the genetics of behavioral traits in dogs.

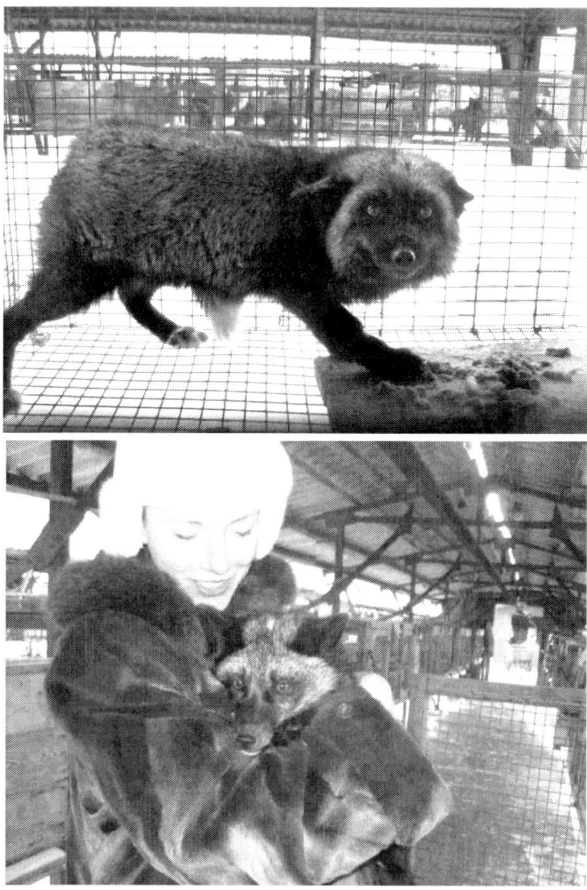

(a)

(b)

Figure 2. Silver fox displaying the wild-type aggressive-avoidance response to humans (a) and silver fox selected for tameness (b) at the Institute of Cytology and Genetics in Novosibirsk. (pictures taken by Darya Schepeleva).

2. Dog History and Domestication

Canine evolutionary history and domestication provide important insights into the genetics of the dog in general and dog behavior in particular. All modern dog breeds are descendants of the grey wolf (Vilà *et al.* 1997; vonHoldt *et al.* 2010). Domestication occurred at least 15,000 years ago (Savolainen, 2007; Vilà and Leonhard, 2007). The process of early canid domestication has been studied experimentally at the Institute of Cytology and Genetics in Novosibirsk (Trut *et al.* 2009). This research group uses silver foxes (*Vulpes vulpes*) as a model for dogs. Silver foxes are taxonomically close relatives of dogs. The experiment started in 1959 with 130 foxes from a commercial fur farm. The foxes were selected for tameness (i.e. lack of fearful or aggressive behavior towards human experimenters) for more than 35 generations at the institute.

The response to human presence was the only selection criterion. The hypothesis was that selection for tameness would lead to development of a domesticated strain of the silver fox. The selection was rigorous: less than 10% of the tamest individuals of every generation were used as parents for the next generation. As a result, offspring displaying aggressive and fear avoidance responses were eliminated from the experimental population in just two to three generations of selection. By the sixth generation, foxes appeared that were eager to establish human contact and exhibited dog-like behaviors such as whimpering to attract attention and sniffing and licking experimenters (Trut *et al.* 2009; Figure 2).

Phenotypic traits that are commonly observed in modern domestic dogs (e.g. loss of pigment, curly tails, drop ears) spontaneously emerged in the fox population selected for tameness (Figure 3).

Behavior and early development thus seem both to be controlled by genes that regulate neural and endocrine systems (Trut *et al.* 2009). An example of such genes could be genes controlling plasma glucocorticoids: cortisol levels in blood of tame foxes were five-fold lower than in the non-domesticated foxes (Trut *et al.* 2009).

In addition, the genes of the serotonergic neurotransmitter system may play a role because alterations in this system were found in the tame foxes (summarized in Trut *et al.* 2009). A recent study of vonHoldt *et al.* (2010) provides another clue about the identity of genes involved in domestication. Their group searched for genomic regions that showed signs of positive selection during early dog domestication using more than 48,000 single nucleotide polymorphisms (SNPs) in dogs and grey wolves. Two out of three genomic regions that were identified have been implicated in memory formation and/or behavioral sensitization in mice or humans (ryanodine receptor 3 and adenylate cyclase 8). They also found evidence for positive selection for a SNP near the *wbscr17* gene. Mutations in this gene result in Williams-Beuren syndrome in humans, which is characterized by social traits such as exceptional gregariousness.

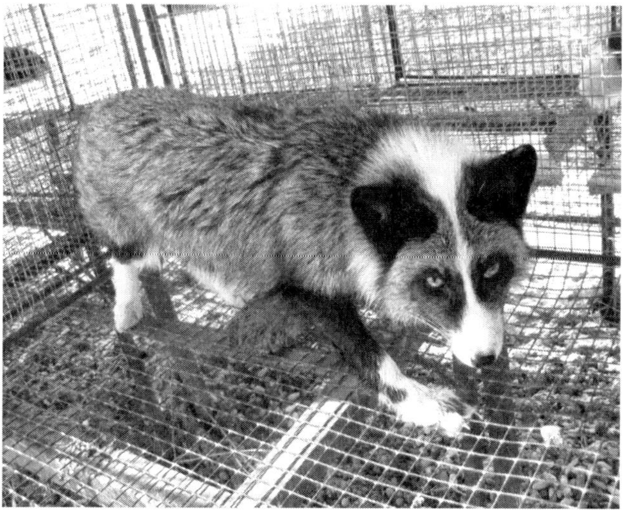

Figure 3. Loss of pigmentation in a silver fox selected for tameness at the Institute of Cytology and Genetics in Novosibirsk. The loss of pigmentation is determined by the homozygous state of the incompletely dominant autosomal *Star* mutation. (picture taken by Darya Schepeleva).

The early domestication was followed by the formation of dog breeds. Various dog breeds already existed in ancient Egypt (Vilà and Leonhard, 2007). However, most of the more than 400 dog breeds that are known today are less than 150 years old. Breeds were often established from a small number of founder dogs. For instance, modern Irish wolfhounds descend from only six founder dogs (Urfer, 2009).

Some breeds experienced severe bottlenecks at times of wars or economic depressions, e.g. only five dogs of the leonburger breed remained alive after World War I. Bottlenecks and small founder populations lead to a so-called "founder effect". When a species invades a new area, the original small population is called a founder population. This term is usually applied in the context of subsequent population growth. Populations with recent founder effects such as the Irish wolfhound and leonburger breeds are expected to exhibit reduced genetic variation due to population bottlenecks. Genetic drift further reduces genetic variation within dog breeds. Genetic drift is the random fluctuation in allele frequencies as genes are transmitted from one generation to the next. Drift is different from selection in that it is a random process, i.e. drift is independent of phenotype. The effect of genetic drift is much stronger in small populations than in large populations. Drift and founder effects can result in a high frequency of risk alleles for diseases.

Many dog breeds have been created by strong artificial selection. Large-effect mutations may become enriched in breeds as a result of the so-called "popular sire effect", i.e. male dogs that have often been used as breeders because of their desired characteristics. Such popular sires may sire more than 100 litters during their life (Ostrander and Kruglyak, 2000). The creation of new breeds within breed groups to enhance certain abilities, e.g. herding or retrieving, or to enhance morphological traits may also impact on breed diversity. During the Victorian era, when many modern dog breeds were created, selection for novelty ("fancy breeds") was popular.

An example is the short-legged phenotype of dog breeds such as dachshund, corgi, and basset hound. The short legs seem to be caused by the expression of a retrogene encoding fibroblast growth factor 4 (*fgf4*; Parker *et al.* 2009). It seems that this shared mutation is the result of historic crosses. In modern dog breeds, genetic homogeneity and the high frequency of risk alleles is maintained by regulated breed barriers: no dog may become a registered member of a breed unless both its parents are registered members of the same breed. There is thus little opportunity for the exchange of genetic material between registered breeds.

The population history described above has led to an enormous inter-breed diversity accompanied by small intra-breed diversity. In other words, dogs of the same breed have highly similar size, morphology, physiology, disease susceptibility, and behavioral characteristics; whereas such characteristics differ substantially between dog breeds. This reflects the enrichment of risk alleles in breeds due to random fixation during bottlenecks, hitch-hiking of mutations near desirable traits and pleiotropic effects of selected variants. As will be explained further in section 3, the canine population genetic history has resulted in a genome that has characteristics that are favorable for molecular genetic studies of complex traits, including a long extent of linkage disequilibrium within breeds and a limited number of short common haplotypes across breeds (Lindblad-Toh *et al.* 2005).

3. The Canine Genome

Before the assembly of the canine genome sequence, linkage analysis in large pedigrees was used to unravel the genetic basis of highly penetrant Mendelian phenotypes in dogs (e.g. Acland *et al.* 1998; Van de Sluis *et al.* 2002). Linkage analysis is not suitable to map risk variants for complex traits such as behavior. The recent assembly of the canine genome sequence and the marker resources that came with it have opened new paths to understanding the underlying genetics of behavior. Having the entire DNA sequence of an organism is now commonplace, but in 2005 the dog was only the fourth species (after human, mouse and rat) to have a full draft assembly of its genome. We had already been given a glimpse of the canine genome with light coverage (1.5 fold) of a poodle named "Shadow" in 2003 (Kirkness *et al.* 2003).

This lighter sequence revealed the DNA sequence similarity of mammals, but it was insufficiently complete to enable researchers to use it to efficiently map genes. The analysis of the full draft (7 fold coverage) genome assembly of a Boxer named "Tasha" (Lindblad-Toh *et al.* 2005) made a more thorough analysis possible. Individual dogs from the same or different breeds were found to differ from one another by only about one DNA nucleotide in every nine hundred (for humans the equivalent figure is 1 in 1,000 nucleotides). So even though they look quite different, individual dogs are genetically very similar. Like humans and mice, dogs have on average about 19,000 protein coding genes. Around 34% of canine DNA exists in sequences that are present in the genome in many copies (these are called retro-transposons or repetitive elements). This number is substantively less than the equivalent values for mouse and human, that are closer to 45% (Lindblad-Toh *et al.* 2005). The domestication of dogs from Grey wolves had been postulated previously (Tsuda *et al.* 1997; Vila *et al.* 1999), but the comparisons made in the canine genome analysis proved beyond question that this was the case.

Tasha's genome revealed for the first time the unique genomic structure of the dog. This structure is the consequence of a close social relationship between dogs and the humans who tended their canine companions and used selective breeding to promote the development of useful behaviors and attractive appearance. The early domestication of dogs from wolves and the later selection of these domesticated dogs into the myriad breeds that we observe today have left indelible marks on the genome.

For example, profound genetic similarity has been observed among dogs from the same breed groupings (Vonholdt *et al.* 2010) and morphological type (Boyko *et al.* 2010) using genome-wide SNP data. The special genomic structure of dog populations greatly enhances our ability to map genetic variants that influence complex traits such as behaviors using the dog. Many geneticists regard dogs as very special indeed.

As part of the canine genome project led by the Broad Institute of Harvard and MIT in Massachusetts, USA (Lindblad-Toh *et al.* 2005), some special ancillary resources were created. The first major ancillary resource was a two million marker SNP map of the canine genome. The creation of this resource enabled researchers to "see" the genetic structure of dog breeds. It had already been observed that dog genomes have marker patterns (haplotypes) that are shared over very long distances, of the order of more than half of a million nucleotides of DNA (Sutter *et al.* 2004).

This is likely to be the result of the bottlenecks, the founder effects and breeding for fancy traits in the breeding history of dogs. Likewise, the genomic researchers were able to see that while the regions of shared haplotypes were very long within dog breeds, across breeds they were quite short, even shorter than for humans. This suggested that special genetic mapping strategies could be employed to exploit this structure.

Mapping genes first within a single dog breed was shown to enable the rapid identification of genomic regions affecting the trait with relatively few dogs and genetic markers required. Then once intervals of association were identified, researchers could move to other related breeds to resolve the regions of association to the level of single genes or even smaller regions within genes and, with this, a high density genotyping array (the next ancillary resource) that would enable the localization of phenotypes to within only a short region of the genome.

Prior to the availability of a complete canine genome sequence, researchers were restricted to trying to link behavior with gene function via inferred information from other species, for example through candidate gene studies. Most frequently, the loci explored were identified through experiments studying known regulatory pathways or mouse knockout experiments. Examples include links with the dopaminergic and serotonergic neurotransmitter systems that are targeted by human psychotropic drugs (van den Berg *et al.* 2005; 2008; Våge *et al.* 2010; Hejjas *et al.* 2007a; 2007b; 2009).

Unfortunately, the candidate gene approach is similar to looking for a needle in a haystack. Aguirre-Hernández and Sargan (2005) have evaluated the candidate gene approach in the study of canine retinal diseases. They reported that only 3.4% of 377 published results of candidate gene studies identified the disease-causing mutation. Therefore, further progress in canine trait mapping is expected with genome wide analyses. In genome-wide analyses there is no *a priori* assumption about which genes are involved in the phenotype. This opens the opportunity for finding genes that have not been associated with the phenotype in question to date.

In addition to genome-wide association studies, alternative mapping strategies have been applied in dogs (Karlsson and Lindblad-Toh, 2008). An example is the development of the CanMap project (Boyko *et al.* 2010), which has highlighted strategies for across-breed mapping in dogs.

By grouping dog breeds with similar phenotypes, the researchers were able to compare breeds to highlight candidate regions of the genome demonstrating signals of selection for the traits of interest. In the CanMap project, the majority of emphasis was placed on aspects of morphological variation, but it is expected that breed-specific behavioral variants will be identified in the near future.

4. Canine Behavioral Genetics

4.1. Heritability of Behavioral Traits

Behavioral genetics is the study of the individual variation of behavior due to genetic differences between persons or animals. The influence of heredity on behavior has been debated for centuries (Plomin, 1990). Genes interact with the environment to determine biological processes in the brain, and as a result, behavior. Environment in behavioral genetics refers to all factors other than inherited factors, e.g. outside temperature, weather conditions, interactions with other animals, training, access to human interaction, diet, hormones, and pathogens. The relative importance of genetic and environmental influences on behavior is a fundamental question in behavioral genetics. Heritability (h^2) is a measure of the relative contribution of additive genetic variance to phenotypic variance (Bourdon, 1997; Nicholas, 2003). Family, adoption, and twin designs have been used to estimate the heritability of human behavioral traits (Boomsma *et al.* 2002; Plomin, 1990). Such studies have shown that there is a significant genetic influence on the majority of human behaviors examined. Heritability estimates for some mental disorders in humans are very high, e.g. 0.90 for autism (Burmeister *et al.* 2008).

Genetic analyses of canine behavior have traditionally been studies of breed differences, selection studies, or population-based heritability studies. Breed differences in behavioral dispositions have been described by many authors (Scott and Fuller, 1965; Svartberg, 2006). The experimental studies of silver foxes at the Institute of Cytology and Genetics in Novosibirsk demonstrate that behavioral traits such as fearfulness and aggression can be manipulated by selection (Trut *et al.* 2009; Figure 2). Foxes that showed dog-like behavior appeared in the sixth generation. This tameness resulted from genetic selection alone because the foxes were not trained (Popova *et al.* 1991). By the 20th generation, 35% of the foxes behaved like dogs. The scientists also succeeded in breeding a colony of foxes with enhanced aggressive behavior (Gulevich *et al.* 2004). These animals were selected for an aggressive and fearful response to the experimenter approaching their cage. The fact that there are breed differences in behavior and that these behavioral dispositions can be selected for, suggests that there is a genetic basis for the individual variation in behavior. Several reviews discuss heritability estimations of behavioral traits in dogs (Houpt and Willis, 2001; Mackenzie *et al.* 1986; Ruefenacht *et al.* 2002). In section 5 of this chapter, we will discuss heritability estimates for specific behavioral traits in more detail. In conclusion, like the studies in humans, research has demonstrated that behavioral tendencies are heritable in dogs.

4.2. Genetic Models

Genes encode proteins that are important for the development and regulation of the neural pathways that regulate behavior. It is believed that many genes with a small effect in combination with environmental influences are involved in the regulation of the normal range of behavioral variation in humans (Plomin, 1990). However, a disruption (e.g. null mutation) of one of these genes can result in a severe deregulation of development. An example of a single gene with a major effect on behavior has been described in a Dutch human family by Brunner and colleagues (1993). Affected male members of this family showed abnormal behavior, including impulsive aggression, arson and attempted rape, as well as borderline mental retardation. The researchers discovered a point mutation in the *MAOA* gene of the subjects. The MAOA enzyme catalyzes the degradation of serotonin, dopamine, and norepinephrine.

The aggressive males produced no MAOA enzyme because the mutation caused a premature stop codon.

Similar to the situation in humans, certain dog families may segregate a genetic variant with a major effect on a behavioral trait, whereas the normal range of behavioral variation in dogs is probably regulated by multiple genetic variants and environmental influences. It should be noted here that Boyko *et al.* (2010) reported that -in contrast to the results from association mapping of quantitative traits in humans – they needed only two to six loci to explain a large proportion (~70%) of the variation in many canine morphological traits such as body size and bone shape. Such a pattern of few quantitative trait loci of large effect has also been observed in other species that experienced recent adaptation and diversifying selection, e.g. the stickleback (Colosimo *et al.* 2004). They explain the finding by the unique population history of the domestic dog, especially the selection for novel traits in the Victorian era. A single mutation could be placed on different genetic backgrounds by crossing various dog breeds. An example is the *fgf4* retrogene that seems to cause short legs in nearly 20 distinct breeds (Parker *et al.* 2009).

Selection for such discrete Mendelian effects is clearly different from the selection methods applied in livestock species, where the population means for economically useful quantitative traits such as milk production, fecundity, and meat quality have been altered by progressive directional selection over many generations. Quantitative selection has acted on subtle individual differences in these traits contributing to the conglomerate phenotype. In livestock the efficiency of this selection has been remarkably enhanced in recent history through the use of sophisticated statistical analysis such as the method of Best Linear Unbiased Predictor (Henderson 1975). Given the complex nature of behavioral traits, we might expect that selection for such traits in dogs has been more akin to traditional selection for quantitative production traits in livestock. If so, we expect that the genetic architecture of canine behavioral traits will have greater complexity than the morphological traits selected by dog fanciers or the Mendelian disorders that have accompanied the increase in inbreeding present in the closed breed populations. Nevertheless, the intrinsically reduced genetic heterogeneity in dog breeds is expected to facilitate the detection of genetic variants affecting behavior in dogs. In addition, it is possible that the severe selection for morphologic traits has resulted in enrichment of variants with large effect that affect behavior through hitch-hiking (Rockman *et al.* 2010).

4.3. Gene-Environment Interactions

In addition to genetic factors, environmental factors also influence behavioral traits. Such environmental factors may include prenatal circumstances such as stress in the pregnant bitch (Serpell and Jagoe, 1995) and early experiences such as maternal care (Scott and Fuller, 1965; Serpell and Jagoe, 1995), living conditions at the home of the breeder (Appleby *et al.* 2002), illness as a puppy (Podberscek and Serpell, 1997; Serpell and Jagoe, 1995), and socialization (Appleby *et al.* 2002; Houpt and Willis, 2001; Scott and Fuller, 1965). Scott and Fuller (1965) demonstrated that the experiences of puppies during the sensitive period (i.e. approximately 3-12 weeks of age) determine which animals and human beings will become their closest social relatives. Some of their experiments involved raising puppies with few human contacts. Such dogs showed extreme fearful behavior and fear-motivated aggression towards humans later in life. Another potential environmental influence is the diet of the dog (DeNapoli *et al.* 2000; Dodman *et al.* 1996; Houpt and Zicker, 2003).

The nature versus nurture debate is outdated. Behavioral genetic researchers agree that behavior is produced by intricate neural networks that are developed and maintained under influence of a variety of genes and environmental factors (Hamer, 2002; Robinson, 2004). Caspi and colleagues (2002) published an illustrative example of gene-environment interaction. They studied a large cohort of male children from birth to adulthood to determine why some children who are maltreated grow up to develop antisocial behavior, whereas others do not. They found a significant gene-environment interaction between a polymorphism of the *MAOA* gene and maltreatment. Maltreated children with a genotype conferring high levels of MAOA expression were less likely to develop antisocial problems.

5. Genetics of Specific Behavioral Traits

5.1. Working Behavior

Dogs were originally selected for working behavior, e.g. guarding, herding, hunting, and pulling sledges. As we mentioned in section 3, the result of this selection can be observed in the canine genome. For instance, Huson *et al.* (2010) observed that the genetic profile of Alaskan sled dogs bred for sprint differs from that of Alaskan sled dogs bred for distance. Many publications present heritability estimates of performance in canine working tests. Examples include in the field behavior test of the Swiss German shepherd dog breeding club (Ruefenacht *et al.* 2002), a hunting behavior test of the Swedish flatcoated retriever club (Lindberg *et al.* 2004), a herding behavior characterization of the Swedish sheep dog society (Arvelius *et al.* 2009), defense competitions in Belgian shepherd dogs (Courreau and Langlois, 2005), and a behavior test for service dogs (Wilsson and Sundgren, 1997a). In most of these studies, a large number of dogs was exposed to a range of standard situations. The behavior of the dogs was scored by trained test leaders. Heritability estimates were mostly low to medium, e.g. between 0.09 and 0.24 in the German shepherd field behavior test (Ruefenacht *et al.* 2002), between 0.1 and 0.4 in the flatcoated retriever hunting behavior test (Lindberg *et al.* 2004), between 0.14 to 0.50 for herding behavior in border collies (Arvelius *et al.* 2009), between 0.07 and 0.18 for defense abilities in Belgian shepherd dogs (Courreau and Langlois, 2005), and between 0.15 and 0.32 for service dog performance (Wilsson and Sundgren, 1997a). For some traits, a higher heritability was found, e.g. "waiting passively in a group" in the hunting behavior test of the Swedish flatcoated retriever club had an estimated h^2 of 0.74 (Lindberg *et al.* 2004).

Chase *et al.* (2009) used an across-breed association method to identify QTLs for several breed stereotypes, including the behavioral traits pointing and herding. SNP data from 147 dog breeds were used in the study. An experienced dog trainer and judge scored the average breed phenotype as qualitative variables, i.e. 0, 1, or NA (Jones *et al.* 2008). The herding QTL (on canine chromosome 1) contains the genes *mc2r* and *c18orf1*. The former is a melanocortin receptor; the latter has been implicated in schizophrenia. The pointing locus on canine chromosome 8 contains the gene *cnih*, which has been implicated in cranial nerve development. However, as the authors also discuss themselves, the across-breed mapping strategy that was employed in this study is sensitive to false positive results due to complex patterns of relatedness between the breeds. Validation of the loci using within-breed segregation analysis is thus required.

5.2. Personality

Personality can be defined as "underlying behavioral tendencies that differ across individuals, that are consistent within individuals over time, and that affect the behavior that is expressed in different contexts" (Stamps and Groothuis, 2010) or "individual behavioral differences that are consistent over time and/or situations (Budaev, 1997). The term "personality" is often used synonymously with "temperament". A study by Svartberg and Forkman (2002) provides insight into canine personality traits. Behavioral data collected using the dog mentality assessment test (DMA) from 1175 dogs of 47 breeds were investigated. The DMA is a standardized behavioral test that consists of ten subtests, during which dogs are exposed to several situations. The test was developed mainly as a tool for breeding of working dogs. The reactions of the dogs were recorded for 33 behavioral variables. The investigators performed factor analysis on these variables and extracted five primary factors: (1) playfulness, (2) curiosity/fearlessness, (3) chase-proneness, (4) sociability, and (5) aggressiveness. Higher order factor analysis showed that all factors except aggressiveness were related to each other, creating a broad factor that influences behavior in a range of situations. This broad factor is comparable to the shyness-boldness axis in humans, which reflects a tendency to approach novel objects and a willingness to take risks (Wilson *et al.* 1994). This broad dimension is supported by earlier dog studies. It was also found to be related to performance in working dog trials (tracking, searching, delivering messages, handler protection): high-performing dogs were bolder than low-performing dogs (Svartberg, 2002).

Svartberg (2006) also performed an analysis of breed differences in personality. DMA data from 13,097 Swedish dogs of 31 breeds were analyzed in this study. Breed scores were calculated for playfulness, curiosity/ fearlessness, sociability, and aggressiveness. The results suggested large differences between breeds in all of the investigated traits, even though there was substantial within-breed variation (Figure 1). Saetre et al. (2006) confirmed the existence of the shyness/ boldness personality trait in the DMA data with an analysis of genetic correlation between the behavioral traits. They estimated the heritability of the behavioral traits using 10 000 German shepherd and rottweiler dogs that performed the DMA. Their results suggest that there is shared genetics behind all behavioral traits except in those related to aggression. Heritabilities were generally low, ranging from 0.04 (remaining fear) to 0.19 (tug-of-war). The heritability of shyness–boldness was estimated to be 0.25 in the two breeds. Ruefenacht *et al.* (2002) have reviewed heritability studies of canine behavioral traits. They report that heritability estimates for traits related to canine personality range from 0 to 0.58 with an average of 0.20.

Several candidate gene studies have attempted to link canine personality traits to specific genetic variations. Heijas *et al.* (2007a; 2007b; 2009) performed a series of candidate gene association studies of the canine dopamine D4 receptor gene (*drd4*). This receptor is abundant in the limbic system of the brain, a region that is involved in emotion and cognitive function. A polymorphism in the human ortholog of *drd4* may be associated with human personality traits and mental disorders including attention deficit hyperactivity disorder (Benjamin *et al.* 1996; Ebstein *et al.* 1997). They studied the *drd4* intron 3 tandem repeat polymorphism in German shepherd dogs using a questionnaire measure of activity-impulsivity (Heijas *et al.* 2007b). The polymorphism was significantly associated with the personality measure in police dogs (n=83), but not in pet dogs (n=55), suggesting a gene-environment interaction (Heijas *et al.* 2007b). They also performed a *drd4* association study using the greeting test, which is based on the DMA (Heijas *et al.* 2009). Ninety-six unrelated German shepherds performed the test, which involved an experimenter approaching and trying to pet the dog. The dog's reaction was coded as follows: 0 points if the dog was not friendly, 1 point if the dog showed friendly behavior but did not follow the experimenter when stepping away, and 2 points if the dog followed the experimenter when stepping away. Higher scores indicate increased interest in novel social companions, which the authors interpret as social impulsivity (Heijas *et al.* 2009). Both the *drd4* intron 3 polymorphism and a polymorphism in intron 2 were found to influence the tendency of the dogs to approach a stranger in a friendly way (Heijas *et al.* 2009). The latter polymorphism was also demonstrated to have an effect on transcriptional activity in luciferase reporter assays (Heijas *et al.* 2009).

Takeuchi *et al.* (2009b) studied 81 Labrador retrievers that were trained as guide dogs. Trainer ratings of the behavior of the dogs were subjected to factor analysis. One of the factors, activity level, was significantly associated with a polymorphism in the solute carrier family 1 (neuronal/epithelial high affinity glutamate transporter) member 2 gene (*slc1a2*) and with a polymorphism in the catechol-O-methyltransferase gene (*comt*). *Slc1a2* encodes a transporter that removes the excitatory neurotransmitter glutamate from the extracellular space. The transporter contributes to the maintenance of low extracellular glutamate concentrations (Kanai *et al.* 1993; Tanaka *et al.* 1997; Trotti *et al.* 1998). Excess glutamate causes neurotoxicity and may contribute to cellular damage in neurologic disorders such as stroke, trauma, Alzheimer disease, amyotrophic lateral sclerosis, and Huntington disease (Choi, 1988; Kanai *et al.* 1993). The *comt* gene has been implicated in human mental disorders including schizophrenia, bipolar disorder, obsessive-compulsive disorder and attention deficit hyperactivity disorder (Craddock et al. 2006).

In conclusion, some preliminary candidate gene associations have been published for canine personality traits. These results require future replication because of the small sample size of the studies. A genome-wide approach to identify genetic variants that influence canine personality traits has been used by Chase *et al.* (2009; see also section 5.1). Their across-breed association study included the personality trait boldness. Like the working traits described in section 5.1, the average breed phenotypes were qualitative variables, i.e. 0, 1, or NA (Jones *et al.* 2008). They identified a locus on canine chromosome 22 which includes the *pcdh9* gene, which encodes a protein localized to synaptic junctions and believed to be involved in specific neural connections and signal transduction. As we discussed in section 5.1, further validation of these results is required.

5.3. Anxiety

Fear is an instinctive natural response to a threat, enhancing an animal's chance of survival. Immediately upon sensing the threat, the nervous and endocrine systems are activated, leading to the classic "flight or fight" response. When faced with a fear-provoking stimulus, a dog's response is governed by: (i) the nature of the stimulus and its importance to the dog, (ii) genetic predisposition, including species-specific behaviors and individual reactivity, (iii) the dog's previous experiences of the stimulus (iv) the perceived effectiveness of various behavioral responses in similar situations in the past. Anxiety is the anticipation of an aversive event. The anticipation of a threat allows the well-adapted animal to avoid the threatening situation. Fear and anxiety produce the same physiological stress response, resulting in a variety of physical and behavioral signs. Physical signs include an increase in heart rate, respiratory rate, blood pressure, salivation and metabolism. Behavioral signs include constant vigilance seen by scanning of the immediate environment, lip licking, yawning, anorexia, vomiting, diarrhea, pacing, crouching, trembling, panting, and grooming.

For the majority of dogs, fear and anxiety are of short duration and increase the chance of escaping danger. For dogs with an anxiety disorder, this state of anxiety lasts much longer. The aversive event may be real or imagined and the dog may become overly sensitive to any perceived threat. A phobia is an extreme fear response, out of proportion to the perceived threat and resistant to habituation. It is the context and the extent of the response that determines if fear and anxiety are reasonable or abnormal.

The most common anxiety and fear disorders seen in dogs are separation anxiety, noise phobias, thunderstorm phobias, and generalized anxiety. In a study examining 1644 canine behavior cases seen at two behavior referral practices over ten years, the prevalence of separation anxiety was 14.4%, generalized anxiety 5.7%, phobias 3.9%, and fears 0.7% (Bamberger and Houpt, 2006). The median age of diagnosis of phobias was 6.5 years compared to 2.5 years for all other behavioral diagnoses, suggesting that learning plays a part in the development of phobias (Bamberger and Houpt, 2006). There is a significant co-morbidity of subtypes of anxiety disorders (Overall *et al.* 2001b). In a study of 141 dogs, animals diagnosed with noise phobia had a probability of 0.88 of suffering from separation anxiety. Dogs with thunderstorm phobia had a probability of 0.86 of also displaying separation anxiety. This co-morbidity is likely the result of a common underlying neurochemical dysfunction.

Anxiety disorders and phobias are maladaptive. Anxious dogs are in a chronic state of apprehension, vigilance and sympathetic arousal. A chronic stress response can contribute to medical problems such as immunosuppression and skin disorders (Seibert and Landsberg, 2008). In production animals, stress has been shown to decrease metabolic efficiency and to reduce reproductive performance (Hemsworth, 2007). It is also reasonable to assume a negative impact on the dog's wellbeing, reducing quality of life, although no reliable measure of this has been established (Stafford, 2008). Anxiety disorders can also interfere with the bond between dog and owner, especially in cases of separation anxiety involving destructive behavior. In addition, anxiety can result in aggressive behavior (Beer *et al*, 2005; Houpt, 2007). Relinquishments and euthanasia are common consequences (Salmon *et al.* 2000).

A genetic component has long been suspected in the development of anxiety disorders. Familial lines of dogs showing extreme "shyness" or "nervousness" have been recognized within many breeds. Scott and Fuller (1965) studied the inheritance of avoidance and vocalization behaviors as an assessment of wildness versus tameness. They found that all basenji puppies showed some fear response during a handling test compared to only 38% of cocker spaniel puppies. When comparing four breeds of dogs (Labrador retriever, German shepherd, Australian kelpie, and boxer), Goddard and Beilharz (1984) found Labradors to be the least fearful.

In the mid 1960s, collaboration between the Neuropsychiatric Research Laboratory of Veterans in Little Rock, Arkansas and the Department of Psychiatry, University of Arkansas established two breeding lines of pointers that were to be maintained for decades (Dykman *et al.* 1966). One line was "susceptible to nervous breakdown", showing an excessive fear reaction to noise, avoidance of humans, freezing catatonic behavior, shivering, reduced exploration, and a slower heart rate. The other line was a stable control population. The lines were raised in an identical environment and subjected to the same behavioral tests. Crosses between the stable lines and the nervous lines consistently produced offspring that closely resembled the nervous strain, especially as regards to avoidance of humans (Murphree, 1973). In the early 1980s, Goddard and Beilharz published several papers on the heritability of canine behavioral traits that determine the suitability of dogs as guide-dogs for the blind. Fearfulness was measured by scoring nervousness, suspicion, sound shyness, and anxiety using a comprehensive behavioral test. It was the most significant cause of failure of potential guide dogs and was estimated to have a heritability of 0.46-0.5 (Goddard and Beilharz, 1982; 1983).

No genetic risk factors for canine anxiety have been identified yet. The serotonergic and GABAergic systems are targeted by many commonly used pharmacological treatments such as tricyclic antidepressants, selective serotonin re-uptake inhibitors and benzodiazepines. Locus coeruleus hyperactivity has been found in humans with panic disorders, with the locus coeruleus producing higher levels of norepinephrine, leading to an over-responsive hippocampus. It seems reasonable to assume that a similar mechanism could be responsible in dogs. A group of 16 dogs with anxiety disorders was found to have a lower serotonin 2A receptor binding index in both the temporal cortex and right occipital cortex compared with normally behaving dogs (Vermeire *et al.* 2009). This suggests that serotonin 2A receptors are involved in the pathophysiology of anxiety disorders in dogs. Results associating the same receptor with panic disorders in humans have been inconsistent, with some finding an association (Inada *et al.* 2003; Unschuld *et al.* 2007) and others not (Rothe *et al.* 2004). A more recent case-control candidate gene association study in humans with panic disorder has implicated serotonin 1A receptors (Blaya *et al.* 2010). With genome-wide association analysis now available, more work can be done to identify candidate genes involved in the development of canine anxiety disorders. Currently research projects are underway across the world to identify genetic variants associated with the development of noise phobias and separation anxiety.

5.4. Aggressive Behavior

Aggression is the most common problem in dogs encountered by behavioral specialists (Landsberg, 2004). Like fear, canine aggression is usually normal behavior (Borchelt and Voith, 1996; Mills, 2003; Mugford, 1984; Reisner, 1997). Wolves use aggression to defend themselves from predators and to compete for food, social status, or reproduction. Situations that elicit aggressive behavior in wolves can also elicit aggression in dogs. Scott and Fuller (1965) observed that the basic patterns of agonistic behavior are similar in dogs and wolves. Agonistic behavior includes behavioral elements such as retreat, submission, and flight in addition to aggressive behavioral elements. However, selection has modified the frequency of expression of agonistic behavior. As a result, dogs and wolves display similar patterns of fighting when sufficiently aroused, but there is a difference in the amount of stimulation required to trigger this reaction (Scott and Fuller, 1965).

There are several kinds of aggression and there are indications that the subtypes have a distinct genetic basis (Houpt and Willis, 2001; Lesch and Merschdorf, 2000; Popova *et al.* 1993; Serpell and Jagoe, 1995; Yeh *et al.* 2010). Aggression can be classified according to assumed motivation (e.g. territorial aggression, redirected aggression) or it can be classified according to target (e.g. owner-directed aggression, dog-directed aggression). Unfortunately, it is not clear which classification of aggression is useful from a genetic point of view. Although canine aggression is usually normal behavior, it can lead to unacceptably dangerous situations (De Keuster *et al.* 2006; Netto and Planta, 1997). Treatment of aggression problems usually involves changing environmental factors through behavioral therapy and sometimes medication is added (e.g. Landsberg, 2004; Overall and Love, 2001a; Reisner, 2003). However, this has limited success and aggression is a common reason for euthanizing dogs (Mikkelsen and Lund, 2000).

Some breeds have intentionally been selected for aggressiveness. For instance, rottweilers, dobermanns, German shepherds, and akitas have been selected for stranger-directed aggression. American pit bull terriers have been selected for fighting purposes (Lockwood and Rindy, 1987). There is ample anecdotal evidence that dog breeds differ in aggressiveness (Lockwood and Rindy, 1987). The results of several studies also provide scientific evidence for breed differences in aggressiveness (e.g. Bradshaw *et al.* 1996; Borchelt, 1983, Blackshaw, 1991, Beaver, 1993; Duffy *et al.* 2008; Hart and Miller, 1985; Landsberg, 1991; Wilsson and Sundgren, 1997b). Scott and Fuller (1965) found breed differences in playful aggression and dominance, with wire-haired fox terriers at the top (i.e. most aggressive) and cocker spaniels at the bottom of the scale. The wire-haired fox terriers developed a large number of dominance relationships before 15 weeks of age, other breeds being slower. They concluded that the terriers were the most aggressive, the basenjis and Shetland sheepdogs next, and the other two breeds the least. The fox terrier puppies also consistently "ganged up" on group members. These attacks were so serious that victims had to be removed in order to prevent serious injury. Svartberg (2006) compared the behavior of 31 breeds using data from the Swedish dog mentality assessment test from 13097 dogs. There were significant differences between the breeds in aggressiveness. We can conclude that there is ample scientific evidence that some breeds have a higher tendency to behave aggressively than others. This is likely to be caused by genetic differences between the breeds. However, it is also obvious from the studies that there is high individual variation in aggressiveness within breeds. This within-breed variance is likely to be partly the result of genetic variation as well.

Twin and family studies in humans suggest a substantial genetic influence on human aggressive behavior, with heritability estimates of approximately 0.50 (Craig and Halton, 2009; Yeh *et al.* 2010). Some early studies of aggression-related traits in police or military dogs failed to produce h^2 estimates higher than zero (Reuterwall and Ryman, 1973; Willis, 1976). However, this is probably due to methodological problems (Houpt and Willis, 2001; Mackenzie *et al.* 1986). Three more recent studies obtained h^2 estimates between 0.06 and 0.33 for aggression scores in behavioral tests (Courreau and Langlois, 2005; Pérez-Guisado *et al.* 2006; Saetre *et al.* 2006). It thus seems that the heritability of aggression is low but significant in the general dog population. However, the heritability of aggression may be much higher in specific dog populations (Liinamo *et al.* 2007).

Two research groups in Japan have studied allelic variation of genes involved in neurotransmission in dogs. A group at Gifu University has published several studies of the above-mentioned canine dopamine D4 receptor gene (Inoue-Murayama *et al.* 2002; Ito *et al.* 2004; Niimi *et al.* 1999). The researchers studied allele frequencies of the polymorphism in 1535 unrelated dogs of 23 breeds. Aggressive breeds tended to have higher frequencies of three specific alleles. However, the behavioral characteristics of the breeds were derived from expert ratings. Such ratings are probably biased. In order to demonstrate an association between the polymorphism and aggression, phenotypes of individual genotyped dogs should be included in the study. In addition, by combining unequal numbers of dogs from breeds with differing allele frequencies, spurious associations are likely to arise.

A few candidate gene studies of canine aggression have been reported. Van den Berg *et al.* (2008) studied four serotonergic candidate genes in golden retriever families segregating aggressive behavior. No evidence for an association of the genes with aggression was found. A genome-wide association study in these dogs resulted in several loci that are currently subject to further analysis (*unpublished results*). Takeuchi *et al.* (2009a) analyzed eight neurotransmitter-related genes in 77 dogs of the shiba inu breed. They reported a significant association between a SNP in the *slc1a2* gene and owner-reported aggression to strangers. The familial relationships between the subject dogs was unknown in this study. The detected association may thus be spurious as a result of familial relationships between the dogs. However, the authors found no significant associations for the other 14 polymorphisms that they studied, increasing the likelihood that the detected association is true. Note that the *slc1a2* gene was also reported to be associated with activity level in Labrador retrievers by the same research group (see section 5.2). In conclusion, no firm evidence for the involvement of specific genetic variants in canine aggression has been presented yet.

5.5. Obsessive-Compulsive Behavior (OCD)

Stereotypes or obsessive-compulsive disorders have been recognized in dogs and have been the subject of research for some time (Luescher *et al.* 1991; Overall, 1998). Canine stereotypical behaviors can manifest as obsessive predatory behaviors such as circling, fence-running, fly or air biting (Overall, 2000), tail chasing (Heywood, 1977; Brown *et al.* 1987; Dodman *et al.* 1993; Schwartz, 1993), or obsessive oral behaviors such as acral lick or blanket sucking (Rapoport *et al.* 1992; Dodman *et al.* 2010). The disorders are first noticed in young dogs around the time of maturity and are most often normal behaviors, but manifested in extreme or inappropriate ways (Overall, 2000). Frequently, in the first instance the behaviors are triggered by environmental stressors. However, the obsessive behaviors soon become habitual and are fixed, often with disastrous consequences for animal welfare (Overall and Dunham, 2002). While the behaviors may be improved with treatment, they are generally regarded as incurable. Obsessive-compulsive behaviors seem to occur more frequently in purebred male dogs. Certain breeds seem predisposed to the disorders. For example, bull terriers frequently exhibit tail chasing, while doberman pinschers are prone to acral licking.

The breed specific prevalence of certain obsessive-compulsive disorders is suggestive of a genetic origin. Studies in other species such as the mouse support this (Overall, 2000). Until the availability of genomic resources for the dog, the genetic underpinnings of these traits remained elusive. In 2010, the first successful genetic mapping of an obsessive-compulsive disorder in the doberman pinscher identified a widely expressed gene responsible for neuronal adhesion, cadherin 2 (*chd2*) as having a significant effect on obsessive behavior. Cadherin 2 is a classical cadherin that is widely expressed, and has a function in left-right axial symmetry and calcium-ion dependent pre-synaptic to post-synaptic adhesion (http://www.nc bi. nlm.nih.gov/omim/ 114020). Dogs showing multiple compulsive behaviors were shown to have a higher frequency of the identified risk allele than dogs with a less severe phenotype (Dodman *et al.* 2010). The study identified a number of genomic signals associated with the trait in addition to *chd2*. Combined with the imperfect Mendelian behavior of the identified locus, this suggests a polygenic causality. Future studies are expected to shed more light on the additional genetic variants involved in this behavior.

5.6. Feeding Behavior

In humans, obesity and its complications are a major health concern in the Western world. Obesity is defined as an accumulation of excessive amounts of adipose tissue in the body. Individual differences in feeding behavior are believed to play a major role in obesity risk (e.g. Nederkoorn *et al.* 2009; Sleddens *et al.* 2008). Such differences in feeding behavior are partly the result of genetic factors. Estimations of the heritability of body mass index (a simple measure of body fat percentage in humans) vary between 0.4 and 0.8 (Walley *et al.* 2009; Wardle *et al.* 2008b). Feeding behavior traits such as satiety responsiveness and food cue responsiveness also have a substantial heritability (De Castro and Lilenfeld, 2005; Llewellyn *et al.* 2010; Wardle and Carnell, 2009). Some of the genetic factors that contribute to this heritability in humans have already been identified (Bauer *et al.* 2009; De Krom *et al.* 2009; Wardle *et al.* 2008a; 2009).As in humans, the prevalence of obesity in dogs is rising in developed countries (Colliard *et al.* 2006; McGreevy *et al.* 2005). Obesity in dogs is often arbitrarily defined as an excess of body weight of more than 15% compared with the ideal body weight (Burkholder and Toll, 2000). It is associated with considerable health risks for the dog (German, 2006; Kil and Swanson, 2010; Zoran, 2010). Owner behavior (i.e. dietary management and offered possibilities for physical activity) seems to play a major role in obesity risk in dogs (Bland *et al.* 2009; Courcier *et al.* 2010). For instance, owners of overweight dogs fed their dogs significantly more treats and exercised their animals less than owners of normal weight dogs according to a questionnaire survey of Bland *et al.* (2009). Owners of obese dogs are also often obese themselves (Kienzle, 1998; Nijland *et al.* 2010).In addition to dog owner behavior, obesity risk is determined by the food preferences and the feeding behavior patterns of the dog. Dogs usually prefer certain foods over others and owners often change food if it seems more acceptable (Houpt and Smith, 1981; Sallander *et al.* 2010). There is also variation in feeding behavior patterns, e.g. some dogs gorge on food whereas others hardly show any interest in food. Food preferences and feeding behavior patterns are the result of the interplay of genetic predisposition, environmental factors and experience. There is anecdotal evidence for breed differences in feeding patterns and food preferences, supporting the genetic contribution to feeding behavior (Bradshaw, 2006; Thorne, 1995). Labradors and pack hounds such as beagles tend to overeat whereas some other breeds are extremely finicky. There is also within-breed variation in food preferences. Breed-differences in obesity risk have been reported frequently (Colliard *et al.* 2006; Edney and Smith, 1986; Jeusette *et al.* 2010; Kronfeld *et al.* 1991; Lauten *et al.* 2001; Speakman *et al.* 2003). Retrievers are consistently found to be more prone to develop obesity in these studies. For instance, retriever breeds had a 4.7-fold increased risk of being overweight compared to other breeds in a study of Colliard *et al.* (2006). Overweight was based on a veterinarian's assessment in this study which included 616 French dogs. The increased obesity risk of retrievers may be a result of metabolic factors, e.g. Labrador retrievers had a lower resting metabolic rate in a study of Speakman *et al.* (2003). However, feeding behavior is also expected to play a role; Labrador retrievers have a reputation for their tendency to gorge.

Genetic factors that influence canine feeding behavior are poorly characterized. One of the genes involved in feeding behavior in other species is the melanocortin-4 receptor gene (*mc4r*). The melanocortin-4 receptor plays a central role in the regulation of energy balance. Activation of the receptor leads to decreased energy intake and increased energy expenditure (Adan *et al.* 2006). Genetic variation at the melanocortin-4 receptor locus (*mc4r*) is associated with body measures and feeding behavior in several species (Bauer *et al.* 2009; Kim *et al.* 2000; Meehan *et al.* 2006; Loos *et al.* 2008; Qi *et al.*

2008; van den Berg *et al.* 2010b). In a preliminary analysis of 187 golden retrievers, van den Berg *et al* (2010a) found no association between *mc4r* polymorphisms and morphological measures in dogs. With genome-wide association analysis available, more work can be done to identify candidate genes for canine feeding behavior.

6. Discussion

6.1. Importance of Behavioral Genetic Studies in the Dog

Dogs fulfill important functions in our society as working partners in military and police organizations, or as farm dogs, assistance dogs, and guide dogs for the blind. In addition, dogs form an important part of our social fabric. They greatly enhance our life experiences as human companions. It has been noted that rapid changes in canine behavioral traits are possible in just a few generations (Svartberg, 2006). This stresses the importance of behavioral considerations in dog breeding programs. The genetics of behavior becomes increasingly important as our societies become more confined and urban. Selective breeding can create better working dogs but can also create better companions in our changing social circumstances.

If we regard behavior as a quantitative/complex trait, it is possible that methods applied in livestock production will have success in canine populations to be selected for behavior. In recent times techniques such as genomic selection have expanded the repertoire of tools available to the breeder to initiate genetic change (Goddard and Hayes, 2007). Genomic selection calculates a genetic score based on the proportion of favorable genetic markers from a genome-wide set shown to be associated with a complex trait of interest. In dog breeding, the application of these technologies would require a coordinated breeding effort on a national or international scale which might be difficult to achieve across the dispersed small holder dog breeding enterprises in most countries. Such small populations, each with different breeding objectives, are likely to be altered more by genetic drift than by the intended selective pressure applied by the breeder (Bulmer, 1972).

6.2. The Dog as a Model for Human Mental Disorders

In humans, evidence for causal associations between specific genetic variants or chromosomal regions and behavioral traits is often inconclusive (Bearden *et al.* 2004; Colhoun *et al.* 2003; Hamer, 2002; Inoue and Lupski 2003). Studying the genetics of behavior using canine models can make important contributions to our scientific understanding of human psychology. Both humans and dogs descend from social species that show cooperative and altruistic behaviors. Many canine behavioral problems resemble human mental disorders that are treated with the same medication (Crowel-Davis *et al.* 2003; Dodman, 1998; Overall 2000). As explained in this chapter, dog breeds are very suitable genetic models for exploring the genetics of behavior. The low genetic heterogeneity within dog breeds implies that only a limited number of the genes that influence a certain behavioral trait will be functionally polymorphic within a breed. This greatly facilitates the chances of finding such genes. The uniformity within breeds is contrasted by the extraordinary variation in behavior between breeds. This combination of intra-breed homogeneity and interbreed diversity provides unparalleled opportunities for elucidating the genetics of behavior. Once we have identified causal mutations in canine genes, it will be interesting to study the involvement of the corresponding genes and proteins in human behaviors.

This has already proven to be a very successful approach for the study of narcolepsy (Chen *et al.* 2009). This disease is characterized by excess daytime sleepiness, striking transitions from wakefulness into rapid eye movement sleep, and cataplexy triggered by positive emotions. It affects 0.02 to 0.18% of the general human population and is a key to understanding other, more common sleep disorders. Familial cases have been reported, but most cases are sporadic. It is considered a complex trait in humans. Some dog breeds also suffer from narcolepsy. The dogs experience cataplexy during vigorous play or when they are excited by being offered their favorite foods (http:// med.stanford.edu/school/Psychiatry/ narcolepsy/moviedog.html). Like in humans, both sporadic and familial cases are observed. Researchers at Stanford University studied a purpose-bred colony of narcoleptic dobermanns and Labradors (Lin *et al.* 1999). Linkage analysis and fine-mapping resulted in the identification of mutations in the hypocretin-2-receptor gene (*hcrtr2)* as causal to the canine disease. Subsequent studies in humans showed that the number of hypocretin-containing neurons in post-mortem samples of the hypothalamus of narcoleptic patients was reduced by 90% (Thannickal *et al.* 2000). It was found that hypocretin might have a key role in circadian clock-dependent alertness. The hypocretin system might be a therapeutic target for more common sleep disturbances in humans.

The more recent research on the *chd2* gene in canine obsessive compulsive disorders promoted excitement among researchers in psychiatric medicine because it suggested new mechanisms for compulsive disorders that might promote better treatment options for humans as well as dogs (Wald *et al.* 2009).

6.3. What's in a Name: Phenotype

It is clear from section 5 that the reliable identification of genetic variants that influence dog behavior is progressing slower than the identification of genetic variants for morphological traits and somatic diseases. One of the reasons for the slow progress of the field of behavior genetics is the difficulty of measuring behavior. As stated by Felix Brown in 1942 "The chief difficulty is to define the condition the heredity of which one is attempting to trace". Correct phenotyping is the key to success of genetic studies (Bearden *et al.* 2004; Mills 2003; Smoller *et al.* 1998). This turns out to be quite difficult in practice in both human and canine genetics. For instance, in our work on the genetics of canine aggressive behavior, we have used three methods for phenotyping: a behavioral test of the dog (van den Berg *et al.* 2003), a questionnaire for the dog owner (van den Berg *et al.* 2006), and a personal interview with the dog owner (van den Berg *et al.* 2003; 2006). We obtained the most promising heritability estimates (i.e. high heritability with low standard errors) for the owner impressions collected during the personal interview (Liinamo *et al.* 2007). This is rather surprising because of the subjectivity of these phenotypes. Jones and Gosling (2005) have reviewed studies of canine personality and noted that "*In theory, test batteries were the closest to achieving objectivity, but in practice the levels of objectivity actually attained varied substantially.*" Large coordinated projects, such as the European LUPA consortium, make an effort to clarify diagnosis by having collaborative organizations follow standard procedures to describe dog temperament (Copeland *et al.* 2008). This is of great value for the progress in canine behavioral genetics.

6.4. Gene Expression Studies

Using genetic association analysis to identify DNA variations that are involved in behavioral differences between dogs is a very useful method for identifying potential causes of normal and abnormal behavior. Another avenue of information can be followed through the observation of the expression of genes in relevant tissues. In our increasingly sophisticated understanding of genomic regulation, we find that non-coding transcripts may play a central role in phenotypic expression (Mattick *et al.* 2010). The analysis of non-coding transcripts has been enabled by the availability of massively parallel sequencing technologies for whole or normalized transcriptome sequencing. Such techniques sample all transcribed sequence in a tissue, not just the coding sequences that have been designed on commercial microarray products.

The high DNA sequence similarity between dogs and wolves suggests that altered gene expression rather than changes in structural gene products may indeed be the main mechanism leading to trait differences between the two species. Saetre and colleagues (2004) compared gene expression in the brains of dogs and wolves. They found significantly altered expression of two neuropeptides, *calcb* and *npy*. They suggested that selection of dogs for behavior during domestication has resulted in changes in mRNA expression patterns of several hypothalamic genes with multiple functions.

Recently, Våge *et al.* (2010) studied the expression of nine genes in different brain regions of eleven dogs that were euthanized because of aggressive behavior and nine non-aggressive dogs euthanized for unrelated reasons using a quantitative polymerase chain reaction approach. The studied brain regions were amygdala, frontal cortex, hypothalamus and parietal cortex, that is, brain areas known for their involvement in emotion. The candidate genes were identified in an initial screening during an earlier phase of the project. Two of the nine genes, *ube2v2* and Zinc finger protein227 (*znf*227) were observed to be differentially expressed in brains of aggressive and non-aggressive dogs. However, these differences were not significant when subjected to multiple testing correction. The *ube2v2* gene is thought to participate in cell proliferation, protein poly-ubiquitination, regulation of DNA repair, regulation of progression through cell cycle, protein modification, and the ubiquitin cycle. *znf*227 is likely to be a transcriptional regulator. From this we may tentatively conclude that genes are expressed differently in the brains of aggressive and non-aggressive dogs, but further work is needed to confirm this finding.

6.5. Breed versus Deed

While the results described in this chapter are promising, much more research is needed before genetic tests can be developed to predict antisocial dog behavior. Governmental legislations for restricted breeds and dangerous dogs have created considerable pressure on animal shelters and animal rescue organizations to employ predictors of aggression risk in dogs (e.g. http://new.dpi.vic.gov.au/pets/domestic-animals/restricted-breed-dogs). There is much debate surrounding the concept of "breed versus deed". Social legislators in many countries restrict ownership or importation of particular dog breeds that are deemed to be dangerous. Home owners in the USA may find difficulty in obtaining home insurance if certain listed breeds are maintained in the household (http://www.bankrate.com/finance/insurance/11-dogs-that-could-raise-your-insurance-costs.aspx). The development genetic tests to predict individual (rather than breed) disposition might be very useful in this debate. However, the heritability of the behavioral traits discussed in section 5 shows that observed behavior in any individual dog is a product of not only its genes, but also its environment (including access to socialization, training, and exercise).

It is thus uncertain whether a reliable molecular test can be developed, even when complete knowledge of the genetics of canine antisocial behavior would be available. In addition, the identification of gene expression patterns that are reliably associated with behaviors may be difficult to apply in practice due to limited access to the tissues of expression in living animals.

A more feasible application of the knowledge of the pathways involved in neuropsychiatric disorders might be the elucidation of drug targets. This could lead to better treatment or prediction of drug efficacy in dogs showing problem behavior.

Conclusion

The synthesis of research carried out into the genetics of dog behavior tells us first and foremost that behavior is substantially inherited in the dog. We know this because different breeds consistently display different characteristic behaviors or susceptibilities to behavioral disorders. In addition, canine behavioral traits have a significant heritability in population-based studies.

Researchers are able to pinpoint the regions of DNA underlying different behaviors efficiently using canine models because of the special structure of the canine genome. Although the identification of genetic variants that affect canine behavior has lagged behind the identification of genetic variants for morphological traits and somatic diseases, the use of such techniques has already led to breakthroughs that have informed research of neuropsychiatric disorders in humans. Such studies have revealed genetic variants with significant influences on behavioral disorders.

The studies have also shown us that behaviors can be complex in their genetic control. Given the substantial heritability of many behavioral traits in the canine, we expect that personality and behavioral traits will be amenable to selection.

This has indeed been shown in the past. Breeders are able to select for dogs with better skills as workers and as better companions in urban communities. Programs aiming for change at a breed level may require coordinated national or international effort.

Acknowledgments

We thank the editors for the invitation to write this chapter.

References

Acland GM, Ray K, Mellersh CS, Gu W, Langston AA, Rine J, Ostrander EA, Aguirre GD. (1998) Linkage analysis and comparative mapping of canine progressive rod-cone degeneration (prcd) establishes potential locus homology with retinitis pigmentosa (RP17) in humans. *Proc. Natl. Acad. Sci. USA*. 95(6):3048-53.

Adan RA, Tiesjema B, Hillebrand JJ, la Fleur SE, Kas MJ, de Krom M. (2006) The MC4 receptor and control of appetite. *Br. J. Pharmacol.*, 149(7):815-27.

Aguirre-Hernández J, Sargan DR. (2005) Evaluation of candidate genes in the absence of positional information: a poor bet on a blind dog! *J. Hered.*, 96(5):475-84.

Akey JM, Ruhe AL, Akey DT, Wong AK, Connelly CF, Madeoy J, Nicholas TJ, Neff MW. (2010) Tracking footprints of artificial selection in the dog genome. *Proc. Natl. Acad. Sci. USA,* 107:1160–65.

Appleby DL, Bradshaw JW, Casey RA. (2002) Relationship between aggressive and avoidance behaviour by dogs and their experience in the first six months of life. *Vet. Rec.,*150:434-38.

Arvelius P, Malm S, Svartberg K, Strandberg E (2009) Genetic analysis of herding behavior in Swedish Border Collie dogs. *J. Vet. Behav.,* 4:237–57.

Bamberger M, Houpt KA. (2006) Signalment factors, comorbidity, and trends in behavior diagnoses in dogs: 1,644 cases (1991-2001). *J. Am. Vet. Med. Assoc.,* 229(10):1591-601.

Bauer F, Elbers CC, Adan RA, Loos RJ, Onland-Moret NC, Grobbee DE, van Vliet-Ostaptchouk JV, Wijmenga C, van der Schouw YT. (2009) Obesity genes identified in genome-wide association studies are associated with adiposity measures and potentially with nutrient-specific food preference. *Am. J. Clin. Nutr.,* 90:951–59.

Bearden CE, Reus VI, Freimer NB. (2004) Why genetic investigation of psychiatric disorders is so difficult. *Curr. Opin. Genet. Dev.,* 14:280-6.

Beaver BV. (1993) Profiles of dogs presented for aggression. *J. Am. Anim. Hosp. Ass.,* 29:564-69.

Beer L, Seksel K, Perry G. (2005) Canine Aggression: An analysis of the frequency of different types seen in a Sydney referral behaviour practice. In: Australian Veterinary Association Conference, Gold Coast, Australia.

Benjamin J, Li L, Patterson C, Greenberg BD, Murphy DL, Hamer DH. (1996) Population and familial association between the D4 dopamine receptor gene and measures of Novelty Seeking. *Nat. Genet.,* 12:81-84.

Blackshaw JK. (1991) An overview of types of aggressive behaviour in dogs and methods of treatment. *Appl. Anim. Behav. Sci.,* 30:351-61.

Bland IM, Guthrie-Jones A, Taylor RD, Hill J. (2009) Dog obesity: owner attitudes and behaviour. *Prev. Vet. Med.,* 92(4):333-40.

Blaya C, Salum GA, Moorjani P, Seganfredo AC, Heldt E, Leistner-Segal S, Smoller JW, Manfro GG. (2010) Panic disorder and serotonergic genes (SLC6A4, HTR1A and HTR2A): Association and interaction with childhood trauma and parenting. *Neuroscience Letters,* 485(1):11-15.

Boomsma D, Busjahn A, Peltonen L. (2002) Classical twin studies and beyond. *Nat. Rev. Genet.,* 3:872-82.

Borchelt PL, Voith VL. (1996) Aggressive behavior in dogs and cats. In Readings in companion animal behavior, V.L. Voith and P.L. Borchelt, eds. (Trenton, New Jersey: Veterinary learning systems), pp. 217-29.

Borchelt PL. (1983) Aggressive behavior of dogs kept as companion animals: classification and influence of sex, reproductive status and breed. *Appl. Anim. Ethol.*, 10:45-61.

Bourdon RM. (1997) Heritability and repeatability. In Understanding Animal Breeding., R.M. Bourdon, ed. (Upper Saddle River: Prentice Hall), pp. 149-84.

Boyko AR, Quignon P, Li L, Schoenebeck JJ, Degenhardt JD, Lohmueller KE, Zhao K, Brisbin A, Parker HG, vonHoldt BM, Cargill M, Auton A, Reynolds A, Elkahloun AG, Castelhano M, Mosher DS, Sutter NB, Johnson GS, Novembre J, Hubisz MJ, Siepel A, Wayne RK, Bustamante CD, Ostrander EA. (2010). A simple genetic architecture underlies morphological variation in dogs. *PLoS Biol.*, 8(8):e1000451.

Bradshaw JW, Goodwin D, Lea AM, Whitehead SL. (1996) A survey of the behavioural characteristics of pure-bred dogs in the United Kingdom. *Vet. Rec.,* 138:465-68.

Bradshaw JW. (2006) The evolutionary basis for the feeding behavior of domestic dogs (Canis familiaris) and cats (Felis catus*). J. Nutr.*, 136(7 Suppl):1927S-1931S.

Brown CJ, Murphree OD, Newton JEO. (1978) The effect of inbreeding on human aversion in pointer dogs. *J. Hered.,* 69:362-5.

Brown SA, Crowell-Davis S, Malcolm T, Edwards P. (1987) Naloxone-responsive compulsive tail chasing in a dog. *J. Am. Vet. Med. Assoc.,* 190(7):884-6.

Brunner HG, Nelen M, Breakefield XO, Ropers HH, van Oost BA. (1993) Abnormal behavior associated with a point mutation in the structural gene for monoamine oxidase A. *Science,* 262:578-580.

Budaev S.V. (1997) "Personality" in the Guppy (Poecilia reticulata): A Correlational Study of Exploratory Behavior and Social Tendency. *J. Comp. Psychol.,* 111:399-411.

Bulmer MG. (1972) The genetic variability of polygenic characters under optimizing selection, mutation and drift. *Genet. Res.,* 19:17-25.

Burkholder WJ, Toll PW. (2000) Obesity. In: Hand MS, Thatcher CD, Reimillard RL, Roudebush P, Morris ML, Novotny BJ, editors. Small animal clinical nutrition, 4th edition. Topeka, KS: Mark Morris Institute.; pp. 401–30.

Burmeister M, McInnis MG, Zöllner S. (2008) Psychiatric genetics: progress amid controversy *Nat. Rev. Genet.,* 9:527-40.

Cadieu E, Neff MW, Quignon P, Walsh K, Chase K, Parker HG, Vonholdt BM, Rhue A, Boyko A, Byers A, Wong A, Mosher DS, Elkahloun AG,

Spady TC, André C, Lark KG, Cargill M, Bustamante CD, Wayne RK, Ostrander EA. (2009) Coat variation in the domestic dog is governed by variants in three genes. *Science,* 326:150–53.

Candille SI, Kaelin CB, Cattanach BM, Yu B, Thompson DA, Nix MA, Kerns JA, Schmutz SM, Millhauser GL, Barsh GS. (2007) A bdefensin mutation causes black coat color in domestic dogs. *Science,* 318:1418–23.

Caspi A, McClay J, Moffitt TE, Mill J, Martin J, Craig IW, Taylor A, Poulton R. (2002) Role of genotype in the cycle of violence in maltreated children. *Science,* 297:851-54.

Chase K, Jones P, Martin A, Ostrander EA, Lark KG. (2009) Genetic mapping of fixed phenotypes: disease frequency as a breed characteristic. *J. Hered.,* 100 Suppl 1:S37-41.

Chen L, Brown RE, McKenna JT, McCarley RW. (2009) Animal models of narcolepsy. *CNS Neurol. Disord. Drug. Targets.,* 8:296-308.

Choi DW. (1988) Glutamate neurotoxicity and diseases of the nervous system. *Neuron,* 1:623-34.

Colhoun HM, McKeigue PM, Davey Smith G. (2003) Problems of reporting genetic associations with complex outcomes. *Lancet,* 361:865-72.

Colliard L, Ancel J, Benet JJ, Paragon BM, Blanchard G. (2006) Risk factors for obesity in dogs in France. *J. Nutr.,* 136(7 Suppl):1951S-1954S.

Colosimo PF, Peichel CL, Nereng K, Blackman BK, Shapiro MD, Schluter D, Kingsley DM. (2004) The genetic architecture of parallel armor plate reduction in threespine sticklebacks. *PLoS Biol.*, 2(5):E109.

Copeland H, Dukes-McEwan J, Sargan D, Kennedy L, Starkey M, Hendricks A, Callanan S. (2008) LUPA - studying human diseases using dog genetics. *Vet. Rec.,* 163:550.

Courcier EA, Thomson RM, Mellor DJ, Yam PS. (2010) An epidemiological study of environmental factors associated with canine obesity. *J. Small Anim. Pract.*, 51(7):362-7.

Courreau J-F, Langlois B. (2005) Genetic parameters and environmental effects which characterise the defence ability of the Belgian shepherd dog. *Appl. Anim. Behav. Sci.*, 91:233-45.

Craddock N, Owen MJ, O'Donovan MC. (2006) The catechol-O-methyl transferase (COMT) gene as a candidate for psychiatric phenotypes: evidence and lessons. *Mol. Psychiatry,* 11:46–58.

Craig IW, Halton KE. (2009) Genetics of human aggressive behaviour. *Hum. Genet.*, 126(1):101-13.

Crowell-Davis SL, Seibert LM, Sung W, Parthasarathy V, Curtis TM (2003) Use of clomipramine, alprazolam, and behavior modification for treatment of storm phobia in dogs. *J. Am. Vet. Med. Assoc.,* 222:744-48.

Cummings JF, de Lahunta A, Braund KG, Mitchell WJ Jr. (1983) Hereditary sensory neuropathy. Nociceptive loss and acral mutilation in pointer dogs: canine hereditary sensory neuropathy. *Am. J. Pathol.,* 112(1):136-8.

Cummings JF, de Lahunta A, Simpson ST, McDonald JM. (1984) Reduced substance P-like immunoreactivity in hereditary sensory neuropathy of pointer dogs. *Acta. Neuropathol.,* 63(1):33-40.

Cyranoski, D. (2010) Genetics: Pet project. *Nature,* 466(7310):1036-8.

De Castro JM, Lilenfeld LR. (2005) Influence of heredity on dietary restraint, disinhibition, and perceived hunger in humans. *Nutrition,* 21(4):446-55.

De Keuster T, Lamoureux J, Kahn A. (2006) Epidemiology of dog bites: a Belgian experience of canine behaviour and public health concerns. *Vet. J.,* 172:482-87.

De Krom M, Bauer F, Collier D, Adan RA, la Fleur SE. (2009) Genetic variation and effects on human eating behavior. *Annu. Rev. Nutr.,* 29:283-304.

De Napoli JS, Dodman NH, Shuster L, Rand WM, Gross KL. (2000) Effect of dietary protein content and tryptophan supplementation on dominance aggression, territorial aggression, and hyperactivity in dogs. *J. Am. Vet. Med. Assoc.,* 217:504-8.

Dodman NH, Karlsson EK, Moon-Fanelli A, Galdzicka M, Perloski M, Shuster L, Lindblad-Toh K, Ginns EI. (2010) A canine chromosome 7 locus confers compulsive disorder susceptibility. *Mol. Psychiatry,* 15(1):8-10.

Dodman NH, Shuster L. (1998) Psychopharmacology of animal behavior disorders. London: Blackwell Science.

Dodman NH, Reisner I, Shuster L, Rand W, Luescher UA, Robinson I, Houpt KA. (1996) Effect of dietary protein content on behavior in dogs. *J. Am. Vet. Med. Assoc.,* 208:376-79.

Dodman NH, Bronson R, Gliatto J. (1993) Tail chasing in a bull terrier. *J. Am. Vet. Med. Assoc.,* 202(5):758-60.

Drögemüller C, Karlsson EK, Hytönen MK, Perloski M, Dolf G, Sainio K, Lohi H, Lindblad-Toh K, Leeb T. (2008) A mutation in hairless dogs implicates FOXI3 in ectodermal development. *Science,* 321:1462.

Duffy DL, Hsu Y, Serpell JA. (2008) Breed differences in canine aggression. Applied Animal Behavior *Science,* 114:441-60.

Dykman RA, Murphree OD, Ackerman PT. (1966) Litter Patterns in the Offspring of Nervous and Stable Dogs: II. Autonomic and Motor Conditioning. *J. Nervous. Mental. Disease,* 141(4):419-32.

Ebstein RP, Segman R, Benjamin J, Osher Y, Nemanov L, Belmaker RH. (1997) 5-HT2C (HTR2C) serotonin receptor gene polymorphism associated with the human personality trait of reward dependence: interaction with dopamine D4 receptor (D4DR) and dopamine D3 receptor (D3DR) polymorphisms. *Am. J. Med. Genet.,* 74:65-72.

Edney AT and Smith PM. (1986) Study of obesity in dogs visiting veterinary practices in the United Kingdom *Veterinary Record,* 118:391-96.

Everts RE, Rothuizen J, van Oost BA. (2000) Identification of a premature stop codon in the melanocyte-stimulating hormone receptor gene (MC1R) in Labrador and Golden retrievers with yellow coat colour. *Anim. Genet.,* 31:194-99.

German AJ. (2006) The growing problem of obesity in dogs and cats. *J. Nut*r., 136(7 Suppl):1940S-1946S.

Goddard ME, Beilharz RG. (1982) Genetic and environmental factors affecting the suitability of dogs as Guide Dogs for the Blind. *Theoretical and Applied Genetics,* 62(2):97-102.

Goddard ME, Beilharz RG. (1983) Genetics of traits which determine the suitability of dogs as guide-dogs for the blind. *Appl. Anim. Ethol.,* 9(3-4):299-315.

Goddard ME, Beilharz RG. (1984) A factor analysis of fearfulness in potential guide dogs. *Appl. Anim. Behav. Sci.,* 12(3):253-65.

Goddard ME, Hayes BJ. (2007) Genomic selection. *J. Anim. Breed. Genet.,* 124:323-30.

Gulevich RG, Oskina IN, Shikhevich SG, Fedorova EV, Trut LN. (2004) Effect of selection for behavior on pituitary-adrenal axis and proopiomelanocortin gene expression in silver foxes (Vulpes vulpes). *Physiol. Behav.,* 82:513-18.

Hamer D. (2002) Genetics. Rethinking behavior genetics. *Science* 298:71-72.

Hart BL, Miller MF. (1985) Behavioral profiles of dog breeds. *J. Am. Vet. Med. Assoc.*, 186: 1175-80.

Hejjas K, Kubinyi E, Ronai Z, Szekely A, Vas J, Miklósi A, Sasvari-Szekely M, Kereszturi E. (2009) Molecular and behavioral analysis of the intron 2 repeat polymorphism in the canine dopamine D4 receptor gene. *Genes. Brain Behav*., 8(3):330-6.

Hejjas K, Vas J, Topal J, Szantai E, Ronai Z, Szekely A, Kubinyi E, Horvath Z, Sasvari-Szekely M, Miklosi A. (2007b) Association of polymorphisms in the dopamine D4 receptor gene and the activity-impulsivity endophenotype in dogs. *Anim. Genet.,* 38:629-33.

Hejjas K, Vas J, Kubinyi E, Sasvari-Szekely M, Miklosi A, Ronai Z. (2007a) Novel repeat polymorphisms of the dopaminergic neurotransmitter genes among dogs and wolves. *Mamm. Genome.,* 18:871-9.

Hemsworth P. (2007) *There is more to welfare assessment than behaviour.* In: Australian Veterinary Association Conference, Melbourne.

Henderson CR. (1975) Best linear unbiased estimation and prediction under a selection model. *Biometrics,* 31:423-47.

Heywood S. (1977) Chasing one's own tail? An example of self-pursuit in a red setter. *Perception,* 6(4) 483.

Houpt KA. (2007) Understanding Anxiety in Cat and Dog Behavior Problems. In: Australian Veterinary Association Conference, Melbourne, Australia.

Houpt KA, Zicker S. (2003) Dietary effects on canine and feline behavior. *Vet. Clin. North Am. Small Anim. Pract.,* 33:405-408.

Houpt KA, Willis MB. (2001) Genetics of behaviour. In The genetics of the dog, A. Ruvinsky and J. Sampson, eds. (Oxon, New York: CABI Publishing), pp. 371-400.

Houpt KA, Smith SL. (1981) Taste preferences and their relation to obesity in dogs and cats. *Can. Vet. J.,* 22(4):77-85.

Huson HJ, Parker HG, Runstadler J, Ostrander EA. (2010) A genetic dissection of breed composition and performance enhancement in the Alaskan sled dog. *BMC Genet.,* 11:71.

Inada Y, Yoneda H, Koh J, Sakai J, Himei A, Kinoshita Y, Akabame K, Hiraoka Y, Sakai T. (2003) Positive association between panic disorder and polymorphism of the serotonin 2A receptor gene. *Psychiatry Research,* 118(1):25-31.

Inoue K, Lupski JR. (2003) Genetics and genomics of behavioral and psychiatric disorders. *Curr. Opin. Genet. Dev.,* 13:303-9.

Inoue-Murayama M, Matsuura N, Murayama Y, Tsubota T, Iwasaki T, Kitagawa H, Ito S. (2002) Sequence comparison of the dopamine receptor D4 exon III repetitive region in several species of the order Carnivora. *J. Vet. Med. Sci.,* 64:747-49.

Ito H, Nara H, Inoue-Murayama M, Shimada MK, Koshimura A, Ueda Y, Kitagawa H, Takeuchi Y, Mori Y, Murayama Y, Morita M, Iwasaki T, Ota K, Tanabe Y, Ito S. (2004) Allele frequency distribution of the canine dopamine receptor D4 gene exon III and I in 23 breeds. *J. Vet. Med. Sci.,* 66:815-20.

Jeusette I, Greco D, Aquino F, Detilleux J, Peterson M, Romano V, Torre C. (2010) Effect of breed on body composition and comparison between various methods to estimate body composition in dogs. *Res. Vet. Sci.*, 88(2):227-32.

Jones P, Chase K, Martin A, Davern P, Ostrander EA, Lark KG. (2008) Single-nucleotide-polymorphism-based association mapping of dog stereotypes. *Genetics,* 179(2):1033-44.

Kanai Y, Smith CP, Hediger MA. (1993) The elusive transporters with a high affinity for glutamate. *Trends in Neurosciences,* 16:365–70.

Karlsson EK, Lindblad-Toh K. (2008) Leader of the pack: gene mapping in dogs and other model organisms. *Nat. Rev. Genet.,* 9(9):713-25.

Karlsson EK, Baranowska I, Wade CM, Salmon Hillbertz NH, Zody MC, Anderson N, Biagi TM, Patterson N, Pielberg GR, Kulbokas EJ 3rd, Comstock KE, Keller ET, Mesirov JP, von Euler H, Kämpe O, Hedhammar A, Lander ES, Andersson G, Andersson L, Lindblad-Toh K. (2007) Efficient mapping of mendelian traits in dogs through genome-wide association. *Nature Genetics,* 39:1321–28.

Kienzle E, Bergler R, Mandernach A. (1998) A comparison of the feeding behavior and the human-animal relationship in owners of normal and obese dogs. *J. Nutr.,* 128(12 Suppl):2779S-2782S.

Kil DY, Swanson KS. (2010) Endocrinology of obesity. *Vet. Clin. North. Am. Small Anim. Pract.,* 40(2):205-19.

Kim KS, Larsen N, Short T, Plastow G, Rothschild MF. (2000) A missense variant of the porcine melanocortin-4 receptor (MC4R) gene is associated with fatness, growth, and feed intake traits. *Mamm. Genome.*, 11(2):131-5.

Kirkness EF, Bafna V, Halpern AL, Levy S, Remington K, Rusch DB, Delcher AL, Pop M, Wang W, Fraser CM, Venter JC. (2003). The dog genome: survey sequencing and comparative analysis. *Science,* 301(5641):1898-903.

Kronfeld DS, Donoghue S, Glickman LT. (1991) Body condition and energy intakes of dogs in a referral teaching hospital. *J. Nutr.*, 121(11 Suppl):S157-8.

Landsberg G. (1991) The distribution of canine behavior cases at three behavior referral practices. *Vet. Med.,* 1011-17.

Landsberg G. (2004) Canine aggression. In Handbook of behavior problems of the dog and cat., G. Landsberg, W. Hunthausen, and L. Ackerman, eds. (Edinburgh etc.: Saunders), pp. 385-426.

Lauten SD, Cox NR, Brawner Jr. WR, Baker HJ. (2001) Use of dual energy X-ray absorptiometry for noninvasive body composition measurements in clinically normal dogs. *Am. J. Vet. Res.*, 62:1295–1301.

Lesch KP, Merschdorf U. (2000) Impulsivity, aggression, and serotonin: a molecular psychobiological perspective. *Behav. Sci. Law,* 18:581-604.

Liinamo A-E, van den Berg L, Leegwater PAJ, Schilder MBH, van Arendonk JAM, van Oost BA. (2007) Genetic variation in aggression-related traits in Golden Retriever dogs *Applied Animal Behaviour Science,* 104:95-106.

Lin L, Faraco J, Li R, Kadotani H, Rogers W, Lin X, Qiu X, de Jong PJ, Nishino S, Mignot E. (1999) The sleep disorder canine narcolepsy is caused by a mutation in the hypocretin (orexin) receptor 2 gene. *Cell,* 98(3):365-76.

Lindberg S, Strandberg E, Swenson L. (2004) Genetic analysis of hunting behaviour in Swedish Flatcoated *Retrievers Appl. Anim. Behav. Sci.,* 88:289–98

Lindblad-Toh K, Wade CM, Mikkelsen TS, Karlsson EK, Jaffe DB, Kamal M, Clamp M, Chang JL, Kulbokas EJ 3rd, Zody MC, Mauceli E, Xie X, Breen M, Wayne RK, Ostrander EA, Ponting CP, Galibert F, Smith DR, DeJong PJ, Kirkness E, Alvarez P, Biagi T, Brockman W, Butler J, Chin CW, Cook A, Cuff J, Daly MJ, DeCaprio D, Gnerre S, Grabherr M, Kellis M, Kleber M, Bardeleben C, Goodstadt L, Heger A, Hitte C, Kim L, Koepfli KP, Parker HG, Pollinger JP, Searle SM, Sutter NB, Thomas R, Webber C, Baldwin J, Abebe A, Abouelleil A, Aftuck L, Ait-Zahra M, Aldredge T, Allen N, An P, Anderson S, Antoine C, Arachchi H, Aslam A, Ayotte L, Bachantsang P, Barry A, Bayul T, Benamara M, Berlin A, Bessette D, Blitshteyn B, Bloom T, Blye J, Boguslavskiy L, Bonnet C, Boukhgalter B, Brown A, Cahill P, Calixte N, Camarata J, Cheshatsang Y, Chu J, Citroen M, Collymore A, Cooke P, Dawoe T, Daza R, Decktor K, DeGray S, Dhargay N, Dooley K, Dooley K, Dorje P, Dorjee K, Dorris L, Duffey N, Dupes A, Egbiremolen O, Elong R, Falk J, Farina A, Faro S, Ferguson D, Ferreira P, Fisher S, FitzGerald M, Foley K, Foley C, Franke A, Friedrich D, Gage D, Garber M, Gearin G, Giannoukos G, Goode T, Goyette A, Graham J, Grandbois E, Gyaltsen K, Hafez N, Hagopian D, Hagos B, Hall J, Healy C, Hegarty R, Honan T, Horn A, Houde N, Hughes L, Hunnicutt L, Husby M, Jester B, Jones C, Kamat A, Kanga B, Kells C, Khazanovich D, Kieu AC, Kisner P, Kumar M, Lance K, Landers T, Lara M, Lee W, Leger JP, Lennon N, Leuper L, LeVine S, Liu J, Liu X, Lokyitsang Y, Lokyitsang T, Lui A, Macdonald J, Major J, Marabella R, Maru K, Matthews C, McDonough S, Mehta T, Meldrim J, Melnikov

A, Meneus L, Mihalev A, Mihova T, Miller K, Mittelman R, Mlenga V, Mulrain L, Munson G, Navidi A, Naylor J, Nguyen T, Nguyen N, Nguyen C, Nguyen T, Nicol R, Norbu N, Norbu C, Novod N, Nyima T, Olandt P, O'Neill B, O'Neill K, Osman S, Oyono L, Patti C, Perrin D, Phunkhang P, Pierre F, Priest M, Rachupka A, Raghuraman S, Rameau R, Ray V, Raymond C, Rege F, Rise C, Rogers J, Rogov P, Sahalie J, Settipalli S, Sharpe T, Shea T, Sheehan M, Sherpa N, Shi J, Shih D, Sloan J, Smith C, Sparrow T, Stalker J, Stange-Thomann N, Stavropoulos S, Stone C, Stone S, Sykes S, Tchuinga P, Tenzing P, Tesfaye S, Thoulutsang D, Thoulutsang Y, Topham K, Topping I, Tsamla T, Vassiliev H, Venkataraman V, Vo A, Wangchuk T, Wangdi T, Weiand M, Wilkinson J, Wilson A, Yadav S, Yang S, Yang X, Young G, Yu Q, Zainoun J, Zembek L, Zimmer A, Lander ES. (2005) Genome sequence, comparative analysis and haplotype structure of the domestic dog. *Nature* 438:803-19.

Llewellyn CH, van Jaarsveld CH, Johnson L, Carnell S, Wardle J. (2010) Nature and nurture in infant appetite: analysis of the Gemini twin birth cohort. *Am. J. Clin. Nutr.*, 91(5):1172-9.

Lockwood R, Rindy K. (1987) Are "Pit Bulls" different? An analysis of the Pit Bull Terrier controversy. *Anthrozoos,* 1:2-8.

Loos RJ, Lindgren CM, Li S et al.; Prostate, Lung, Colorectal, and Ovarian (PLCO) Cancer Screening Trial; KORA; Nurses' Health Study; Diabetes Genetics Initiative; SardiNIA Study; Wellcome Trust Case Control Consortium; FUSION. (2008) Common variants near MC4R are associated with fat mass, weight and risk of obesity. *Nat. Genet.,* 40:768–75.

Luescher UA, McKeown DB, Halip J. (1991) Stereotypic or obsessive-compulsive disorders in dogs and cats. *Vet. Clin. North Am. Small Anim. Pract.,* 21(2):401-13.

Mackenzie SA, Oltenacu EAB, Houpt KA. (1986) Canine Behavioral Genetics – a Review. *Appl. Anim. Behav. Sci.,* 15, 365-93.

Mattick JS, Taft RJ, Faulkner GJ. (2010) A global view of genomic information--moving beyond the gene and the master regulator. *Trends Genet.,* 26:21-8.

McGreevy PD, Thomson PC, Pride C, Fawcett A, Grassi T, Jones B. (2005) Prevalence of obesity in dogs examined by Australian veterinary practices and the risk factors involved. *Vet. Rec.*, 156:695–707.

Meehan TP, Tabeta K, Du X, Woodward LS, Firozi K, Beutler B, Justice MJ. (2006) Point mutations in the melanocortin-4 receptor cause variable obesity in mice.*Mamm. Genome,* 17:1162–71.

Mikkelsen J, Lund JD. (2000) Euthanasia of dogs due to behavioural problems: an epidemiological study of euthanasia of dogs in Denmark, with a special focus on problems of aggression. *Eur. J. Comp. Anim. Pract., X,* 143-50.

Mills DS. (2003) Medical paradigms for the study of problem behaviour: a critical review. *Appl. Anim. Behav. Sci.,* 81:265-77.

Mugford RA. (1984) Behaviour problems in the dog. In Nutrition and behaviour in dogs and cats., R.S. Anderson, ed. (Oxford, etc.: Pergamon Press), pp. 207-15.

Murphree OD. (1973) Inheritance of Human Avoidance and Inactivity in Two Strains of the Pointer Dog. *Biological Psychiatry,* 7(1):23-9.

Nederkoorn C, Guerrieri R, Havermans RC, Roefs A, Jansen A. (2009) The interactive effect of hunger and impulsivity on food intake and purchase in a virtual supermarket. *Int. J. Obes. (Lond),* 33(8):905-12.

Netto WJ, Planta DJU. (1997) Behavioural testing for aggression in the domestic dog. *Appl. Anim. Behav. Sci.,* 52:243-63.

Nicholas FW. (2003) Quantitative variation. In *Introduction to veterinary genetics.,* F.W. Nicholas, ed. (Oxford: Blackwell Publishing), pp. 191-201.

Nijland ML, Stam F, Seidell JC. (2010) Overweight in dogs, but not in cats, is related to overweight in their owners. *Public Health Nutrition:* 13(1):102–6.

Niimi Y, Inoue-Murayama M, Murayama Y, Ito S, Iwasaki T. (1999) Allelic variation of the D4 dopamine receptor polymorphic region in two dog breeds, Golden retriever and Shiba. *J Vet. Med. Sci.,* 61:1281-86.

Ostrander EA, Kruglyak L. (2000) Unleashing the canine genome. *Genome Research,* 10:1271-74.

Overall KL. (1998) Concerns regarding study of obsessive-compulsive disorder in dogs. *J. Am. Vet. Med. Assoc.,* 213(2):198-9.

Overall KL. (2000) Natural animal models of human psychiatric conditions: assessment of mechanism and validity. *Prog. Neuropsychopharmacol Biol. Psychiatry,* 24(5):727-76.

Overall KL, Dunham AE, Frank D. (2001b) Frequency of nonspecific clinical signs in dogs with separation anxiety, thunderstorm phobia, and noise phobia, alone or in combination. *Journal of the American Veterinary Medical Association,* 219(4):467-73.

Overall KL, Love M. (2001a) Dog bites to humans--demography, epidemiology, injury, and risk. *J. Am. Vet. Med. Assoc,,* 218:1923-34.

Overall KL, Dunham AE. (2002) Clinical features and outcome in dogs and cats with obsessive-compulsive disorder: 126 cases (1989-2000). *J. Am. Vet. Med. Assoc.*, 221(10): 1445-52.

Paradis M, de Jaham C, Page N, Sauve F, Helie P. (2005). Acral mutilation and analgesia in 13 French spaniels. *Vet. Dermatol.*, 16(2):87-93.

Parker HG, VonHoldt BM, Quignon P, Margulies EH, Shao S, Mosher DS, Spady TC, Elkahloun A, Cargill M, Jones PG, Maslen CL, Acland GM, Sutter NB, Kuroki K, Bustamante CD, Wayne RK, Ostrander EA. (2009) An expressed fgf4 retrogene is associated with breed-defining chondrodysplasia in domestic dogs. *Science*, 325(5943):995-8.

Parker HG, Sutter NB, Ostrander EA. (2006) Understanding Genetic Relationships among Purebred Dogs: The PhyDo Project. In Ostrander EA, Giger U, Lindblad-Toh K. (eds) *The dog and its genome*. New York: Cold Spring Harbor Laboratory Press 141-157.

Pérez-Guisado J, Lopez-Rodríguez R, Muñoz-Serrano A. (2006) Heritability of dominant–aggressive behaviour in English Cocker Spaniels. *Appl. Anim. Behav. Sci.*, 100:219-27

Plomin R. (1990) *Nature and nurture: an introduction to human behavioral genetics*. (Pacific Grove, California: Brooks/Cole).

Podberscek AL, Serpell JA. (1997) Environmental influences on the expression of aggressive behaviour in English Cocker Spaniels. *Appl. Anim. Behav. Sci.*, 52:215-27.

Popova NK, Nikulina EM, Kulikov AV. (1993) Genetic analysis of different kinds of aggressive behavior. *Behav. Genet.*, 23:491-97.

Popova NK, Voitenko NN, Kulikov AV, Avgustinovich DF. (1991) Evidence for the involvement of central serotonin in mechanism of domestication of silver foxes. *Pharmacol. Biochem. Behav.*, 40:751-56.

Qi L, Kraft P, Hunter DJ, Hu FB. (2008) The common obesity variant near MC4R gene is associated with higher intakes of total energy and dietary fat, weight change and diabetes risk in women. *Hum. Mol. Genet.*, 17:3502–08.

Rapoport JL, Ryland DH, Kriete M. (1992) Drug treatment of canine acral lick. An animal model of obsessive-compulsive disorder. *Arch. Gen. Psychiatry,* 49(7):517-21.

Reisner IR. (1997) Assessment, management, and prognosis of canine dominance-related aggression. *Vet. Clin. North Am. Small Anim. Pract.,* 27:479-95.

Reisner IR. (2003) Differential diagnosis and management of human-directed aggression in dogs. *Vet. Clin. North Am. Small Anim. Pract.*, 33:303-20.

Reuterwall C, Ryman N. (1973) An estimate of the magnitude of additive genetic variation of some mental characters in Alsatian dogs. *Hereditas,* 73:277-84.

Robinson GE. (2004) Genomics. Beyond nature and nurture. *Science,* 304:397-99.

Rockman MV, Skrovanek SS, Kruglyak L. (2010) Selection at linked sites shapes heritable phenotypic variation in C. elegans. *Science*, 330:372-6.

Rothe C, Koszycki D, Bradwejn J, King N, De Luca V, Shaikh S, Franke P, Garritsen H, Fritze J, Deckert J, Kennedy JL. (2004) Association study of serotonin-2A receptor gene polymorphism and panic disorder in patients from Canada and Germany. *Neuroscience Letters,* 363(3):276-79.

Ruefenacht S, Gebhardt-Henrich S, Miyake T, Gaillard C. (2002) A behaviour test on German Shepherd dogs: heritability of seven different traits *Applied Animal Behaviour Science* ,79:113-32.

Saetre P, Strandberg E, Sundgren PE, Pettersson U, Jazin E, Bergström TF. (2006) The genetic contribution to canine personality. *Genes. Brain Behav.*, 5(3):240-8.

Sallander M, Hagberg M, Hedhammar A, Rundgren M, Lindberg JE. (2010) Energy-intake and activity risk factors for owner-perceived obesity in a defined population of Swedish dogs. *Prev. Vet. Med.*, 1; 96(1-2):132-41.

Salmon, M. D., J. Hutchison, et al. (2000) Behavioral Reasons for Relinquishment of Dogs and Cats to 12 Shelters. *J. Appl. Anim. Welfare. Sci.,* 3(2):93-106.

Salmon Hillbertz NH, Isaksson M, Karlsson EK, Hellmén E, Pielberg GR, Savolainen P, Wade CM, von Euler H, Gustafson U, Hedhammar A, Nilsson M, Lindblad-Toh K, Andersson L, Andersson G. (2007) Duplication of FGF3, FGF4, FGF19 and ORAOV1 causes hair ridge and predisposition to dermoid sinus in Ridgeback dogs. *Nature Genetics,* 39:1318–20.

Savolainen (2007) Domestication of dogs. In Jensen P. (ed.) *The behavioral biology of dogs*. Oxfordshire UK: CABI, pp 21-37.

Scherrer JF, True WR, Xian H, Lyons MJ, Eisen SA, Goldberg J, Lin N, Tsuang MT. (2000) Evidence for genetic influences common and specific to symptoms of generalized anxiety and panic. *Journal of Affective Disorders,* 57(1-3):25-35.

Schwartz S. (1993) Naltrexone-induced pruritus in a dog with tail-chasing behavior. *J. Am. Vet. Med. Assoc.,* 202(2):278-80.

Scott JP, Fuller JL. (1965) Genetics and the Social Behavior of the Dog. Chicago, The University of Chicago Press.

Seibert LM, Landsberg GM. (2008) Diagnosis and Management of Patients Presenting with Behavior Problems. *Veterinary Clinics of North America: Small Animal Practice,* 38(5): 937-50.

Serpell JA, Jagoe JA. (1995) Early experience and the development of behaviour. In The Domestic dog: its evolution, behaviour, and interactions with people., *J. Serpell*, ed. (Cambridge: Cambridge University Press), pp. 79-102.

Sleddens EFC, Kremers SPJ, Thijs C. (2008) The Children's Eating Behaviour Questionnaire: factorial validity and association with Body Mass Index in Dutch children aged 6-7. *Int. J. Behav. Nutr. Phys. Activity,* 5:49-57.

Spady TC, Ostrander EA. (2008) Canine behavioral genetics: pointing out the phenotypes and herding up the genes. *Am. J. Hum. Genet.*, 82(1):10-8.

Speakman, J.R., van Acker, A., Harper, E.J. (2003) Age-related changes in the metabolism and body composition of three dog breeds and their relationship to life expectancy. *Aging Cell*, 2:265–75.

Stafford K. (2008) *How Behavioural Problems Influence the Welfare of Dogs*. In: 33rd World Small Animal Veterinary Congress, Dublin, Ireland.

Stamps J, Groothuis TGG. (2010) The development of animal personality: relevance, concepts and perspectives. *Biol. Rev.,* 85:301-25.

Sutter NB, Bustamante CD, Chase K, Gray MM, Zhao K, Zhu L, Padhukasahasram B, Karlins E, Davis S, Jones PG, Quignon P, Johnson GS, Parker HG, Fretwell N, Mosher DS, Lawler DF, Satyaraj E, Nordborg M, Lark KG, Wayne RK, Ostrander EA. (2007) A single IGF1 allele is a major determinant of small size in dogs. *Science,* 316:112–15.

Sutter NB, Eberle MA, Parker HG, Pullar BJ, Kirkness EF, Kruglyak L, Ostrander EA. (2004) Extensive and breed-specific linkage disequilibrium in Canis familiaris. *Genome. Res.,* 14(12):2388-96.

Svartberg K. (2006) Breed-typical behaviour in dogs - Historical remnants or recent constructs? *Appl. Anim. Behav. Sci.,* 96:293-313.

Svartberg K, Forkman B. (2002) Personality traits in the domestic dog (Canis familiaris). *Appl. Anim. Behav. Sci.,* 79:133-55.

Svartberg K. (2002) Shyness-boldness predicts performance in working dogs *Appl. Anim. Behav. Sci*., 79:157–74.

Takeuchi Y, Hashizume C, Arata S, Inoue-Murayama M, Maki T, Hart BL, Mori Y. (2009b) An approach to canine behavioural genetics employing guide dogs for the blind. *Anim. Genet.*, 40(2):217-24.

Takeuchi Y, Kaneko F, Hashizume C, Masuda K, Ogata N, Maki T, Inoue-Murayama M, Hart BL, Mori Y. (2009a) Association analysis between canine behavioural traits and genetic polymorphisms in the Shiba Inu breed. *Anim. Genet.*, 40(5):616-22.

Tanaka K, Watase K, Manabe T, Yamada K, Watanabe M, Takahashi K, Iwama H, Nishikawa T, Ichihara N, Kikuchi T, Okuyama S, Kawashima N, Hori S, Takimoto M, Wada K. (1997) Epilepsy and exacerbation of brain injury in mice lacking the glutamate transporter GLT-1. *Science,* 276:1699–702.

Thannickal TC, Moore RY, Nienhuis R, Ramanathan L, Gulyani S, Aldrich M, Cornford M, Siegel JM. (2000) Reduced number of hypocretin neurons in human narcolepsy. *Neuron*, 27(3):469-74.

Thorne C. (1995) Feeding behaviour of domestic dogs and the role of experience. In The domestic dog- its evolution, behaviour and interactions with people, J. Serpell, ed. (Cambridge: Cambridge University Press), pp. 104-114.

Trotti D, Danbolt NC, Volterra A. (1998) Glutamate transporters are oxidant-vulnerable: a molecular link between oxidative and excitotoxic neurodegeneration? *Trends Pharmacol Sci.,* 19(8):328-34.

Trut L, Oskina I, Kharlamova A. (2009) Animal evolution during domestication: the domesticated fox as a model. *Bioessays.*, 31(3):349-60.

Tsuda K, Kikkawa Y, Yonekawa H, Tanabe Y. (1997) Extensive interbreeding occurred among multiple matriarchal ancestors during the domestication of dogs: evidence from inter- and intraspecies polymorphisms in the D-loop region of mitochondrial DNA between dogs and wolves. *Genes Genet. Syst.,* 72(4):229-38.

Unschuld PG, Ising M, Erhardt A, Lucae S, Kloiber S, Kohli M, Salyakina D, Welt T, Kern N, Lieb R, Uhr M, Binder EB, Müller-Myhsok B, Holsboer F, Keck ME. (2007) Polymorphisms in the serotonin receptor gene HTR2A are associated with quantitative traits in panic disorder. *Amn. J. Med. Genet., B: Neuropsychiatric Genetics* 144B(4):424-29.

Urfer SR. (2009) Inbreeding and fertility in Irish Wolfhounds in Sweden: 1976 to 2007. *Acta. Vet. Scand.*, 51:21.

Våge J, Wade C, Biagi T, Fatjó J, Amat M, Lindblad-Toh K, Lingaas F. (2010) Association of dopamine- and serotonin-related genes with canine aggression. *Genes. Brain Behav.,* 9, 372-8.

Van de Sluis B, Rothuizen J, Pearson PL, van Oost BA, Wijmenga C. (2002) Identification of a new copper metabolism gene by positional cloning in a purebred dog population. *Hum. Mol. Genet.*, 11:165–73

Van den Berg SM, Heuven HC, van den Berg L, Duffy DL, Serpell JA. (2010c) Measuring stranger-directed aggression in three common dog breeds. *Applied Animal Behaviour Science,* 124:136–41.

Van den Berg L, van Beekum O, Heutink P, Felius B, van de Heijning M, Strijbis S, van Spaendonk R, Piancatelli D, Garner KM, El Aouad R, Sistermans E, Adan RAH, Delemarre-van de Waal HA. (2010b) Melanocortin-4 receptor gene mutations in a Dutch cohort of obese children *Obesity (Silver Spring).* 2010 Oct 21. [Epub ahead of print] PMID: 20966905.

Van den Berg L, van den Berg S, Martens EECP, Hazewinkel HAW, Dijkshoorn NA, Delemarre-van de Waal HA, Heutink P, Leegwater PAJ, Heuven HCM. (2010a) Analysis of Variation in the Melanocortin-4 Receptor Gene (mc4r) in Golden Retriever Dogs. *Animal Genetics,* 41:557–60.

Van den Berg L, Vos-Loohuis M, Schilder MBH, van Oost BA, Hazewinkel HAW, Wade CM, Karlsson EK, Lindblad-Toh K, Liinamo A-E, Leegwater PAJ. (2008) Evaluation of the serotonergic genes htr1A, htr1B, htr2A, and slc6A4 in aggressive behavior of Golden Retriever dogs. *Behavior Genetics,* 38:55-66.

Van den Berg L, Schilder MB, de Vries H, Leegwater PA, van Oost BA. (2006) Phenotyping of aggressive behavior in golden retriever dogs with a questionnaire. *Behav. Genet.*, 36:882-902.

Van den Berg L, Kwant L, Hestand MS, van Oost BA, Leegwater PAJ. (2005) Structure and variation of three canine genes involved in serotonin binding and transport: the serotonin receptor 1A gene (htr1A), serotonin receptor 2A gene (htr2A), and serotonin transporter gene (slc6A4). *J. Hered.,* 96:786-96.

Van den Berg L, Schilder MBH, Knol BW. (2003) Behavior genetics of canine aggression: behavioral phenotyping of golden retrievers by means of an aggression test. *Behavior Genetics,* 33:469-83.

Vermeire ST, Audenaert KR, Dobbeleir AA, De Meester RH, De Vos FJ, Peremans KY. (2009) Evaluation of the Brain 5-HT2A Receptor Binding Index in Dogs with Anxiety Disorders, Measured with 123I-5I-R91150 and SPECT. *J. Nucl. Med.,* 50(2):284-89.

Vilà C, Maldonado JE, Wayne RK. (1999) Phylogenetic relationships, evolution, and genetic diversity of the domestic dog. *J. Hered.,* 90(1):71-7.

Vilà C, Leonhard (2007). Origin of breed diversity. In Jensen P. (ed.) The behavioral biology of dogs. Oxfordshire UK: CABI, pp 21-37.

Vilà C, Savolainen P, Maldonado JE, Amorim IR, Rice JE, Honeycutt RL, Crandall KA, Lundeberg J, Wayne RK. (1997) Multiple and ancient origins of the domestic dog. *Science,* 276:1687-89.

Vonholdt BM, Pollinger JP, Lohmueller KE, Han E, Parker HG, Quignon P, Degenhardt JD, Boyko AR, Earl DA, Auton A, Reynolds A, Bryc K, Brisbin A, Knowles JC, Mosher DS, Spady TC, Elkahloun A, Geffen E, Pilot M, Jedrzejewski W, Greco C, Randi E, Bannasch D, Wilton A, Shearman J, Musiani M, Cargill M, Jones PG, Qian Z, Huang W, Ding ZL, Zhang YP, Bustamante CD, Ostrander EA, Novembre J, Wayne RK. (2010) Genome-wide SNP and haplotype analyses reveal a rich history underlying dog domestication. *Nature*, 464(7290):898-902.

Wald R, Dodman N, Shuster L. (2009) The combined effects of memantine and fluoxetine on an animal model of obsessive compulsive disorder. *Exp. Clin. Psychopharmacol.,* 17(3): 191-7.

Walley AJ, Asher JE, Froguel P. (2009) The genetic contribution to non-syndromic human obesity. *Nat. Rev. Genet.*, 10:431-42.

Wardle J, Llewellyn C, Sanderson S, Plomin R. (2009) The FTO gene and measured food intake in children. *Int. J. Obes., (Lond).* 33(1):42-5.

Wardle J, Carnell S. (2009) Appetite is a Heritable Phenotype Associated with Adiposity. *Ann Behav Med.* 2009 Sep 3; PMID: 19730964.

Wardle J, Carnell S, Haworth CM, Farooqi IS, O'Rahilly S, Plomin R. (2008a) Obesity associated genetic variation in FTO is associated with diminished satiety. *J. Clin. Endocrinol. Metab.*, 93:3640-3.

Wardle J, Carnell S, Haworth CM, Plomin R. (2008b) Evidence for a strong genetic influence on childhood adiposity despite the force of the obesogenic environment. *Am. J. Clin. Nutr.*, 87:398-404.

Wardle J, Guthrie C, Sanderson S, Birch L, Plomin R. (2001) Food and activity preferences in children of lean and obese parents. *Int. J. Obes. Relat. Metab. Disord.*, 25(7):971-7.

Willis MB. (1976) The German Shepherd Dog - Its History, Development and Genetics. (Leicestor, UK: K.andR. Books).

Wilsson E, Sundgren P-E. (1997a) The use of a behaviour test for the selection of dogs for service and breeding, II: Heritability for tested parameters and effect of selection based on service dog characteristics. *Appl. Anim. Behav. Sci.*, 54:235-41.

Wilsson E, Sundgren P-E. (1997b) The use of a behaviour test for the selection of dogs for service and breeding, I: Method of testing and evaluating test results in the adult dog, demands on different kinds of service dogs, sex and breed differences. *Appl. Anim. Behav. Sci.,* 53:279-95.

Wilson D, Clark A, Coleman K, Dearstyne T. (1994) Shyness and boldness in humans and other animals. *Trends Ecol. Evol.,* 9:442–46.

Yeh MT, Coccaro EF, Jacobson KC. (2010) Multivariate behavior genetic analyses of aggressive behavior subtypes. *Behav. Genet.*, 40(5):603-17.

Zoran DL. (2010) Obesity in dogs and cats: a metabolic and endocrine disorder. *Vet. Clin. North Am. Small Anim. Pract.,* 40(2):221-39.

Index

D

E

F

G

H

N

Q

R

S

T

U

V